Disclaimer and/or Legal Notices:

CONTENTS

UNVEILING THE HIDDEN HEALING SECRETS OF THE SCRIPTURES

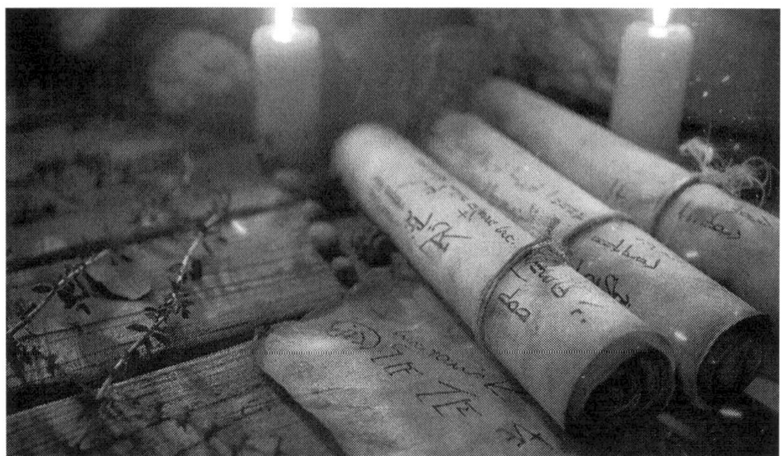

What if the ultimate health manual has been hiding in plain sight for centuries? The Bible, revered as a spiritual compass, also holds profound principles for physical health and well-being—principles that modern medicine is only now beginning to validate. These ancient truths are more than just symbolic; they offer practical, transformative guidance for anyone seeking vitality, longevity, and peace.

Throughout the Bible, we see evidence of God's wisdom in health, from dietary laws to instructions for rest and renewal. Yet these teachings often go unnoticed in a world captivated by fleeting health trends and quick fixes. This book seeks to shine a light on the overlooked biblical principles that can revolutionize your approach to health.

HEALING MIRACLES THAT PROVE GOD'S POWER

The Gospels are brimming with stories of miraculous healings—evidence of God's power to restore broken bodies and spirits. Jesus healed the sick, gave sight to the blind, and even raised the dead. These miracles weren't just acts of compassion; they were demonstrations of the divine power to heal and renew. But what if these stories hold lessons for us today, guiding us toward a deeper understanding of health that integrates faith and action? As we explore these miracles, we'll uncover their relevance to modern health challenges and the timeless principles they reveal.

<u>**WHY MODERN LIFESTYLES IGNORE DIVINE WISDOM**</u>

In our fast-paced, technology-driven world, we've drifted from the rhythms and practices God designed for our flourishing. Processed foods, sedentary lifestyles, and chronic stress dominate our lives, leaving us physically and spiritually depleted. By contrast, the Bible teaches the importance of balance, rest, and living in harmony with God's creation. This book will expose the ways modern lifestyles undermine our health and show you how to realign with divine wisdom to experience renewal.

<u>**YOUR JOURNEY TO RECLAIMING BIBLICAL HEALTH**</u>

This isn't just a book—it's an invitation to transformation. The journey ahead is about more than reclaiming physical health; it's about restoring your connection to God and His design for your life. By embracing biblical principles, you'll discover a path to health that nourishes your body, mind, and spirit. From ancient dietary practices to the spiritual discipline of fasting, from natural remedies to the healing power of gratitude, you'll be equipped with tools to embark on a journey of profound renewal.

The time has come to rediscover the healing secrets God has placed in His Word. These truths aren't relics of the past; they are living, powerful principles that can change your life today. Are you ready to reclaim the vibrant health God intended for you? Let the journey begin.

THE ANCIENT EDEN DIET FOR PERFECT HEALTH

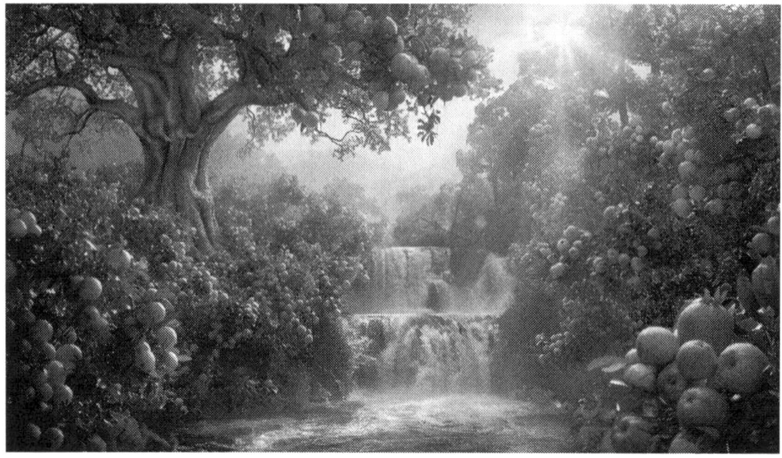

Imagine a time before disease, stress, or exhaustion—a time when humanity lived in perfect harmony with creation. The Garden of Eden wasn't just a place of spiritual connection; it was the blueprint for a life of perfect health. At the heart of this design was a diet crafted by God Himself, one centered on seed-bearing plants, fruits, and herbs. This wasn't just food; it was nourishment imbued with divine intention, designed to sustain the body, mind, and spirit in flawless balance.

Today, we've drifted far from this Edenic ideal. Processed foods and artificial additives have replaced the pure, life-giving nourishment of God's creation. But the secrets of the Eden diet are still accessible. Modern science is now uncovering the extraordinary health benefits of these ancient superfoods, from the antioxidants in pomegranates to the healing properties of figs and herbs. By returning to the foods God provided in the beginning, we can unlock a vibrant, energized life and rediscover the health that was always meant to be ours.

DISCOVER THE SUPERFOODS GOD DESIGNED FOR YOU

From the very first chapter of Genesis, God revealed a powerful truth: the foods He provided were meant to sustain not just life but abundant health. In Genesis 1:29, He says, "I give you every seed-bearing plant on the face of the whole earth and every tree that has fruit with seed in it. They will be yours for food." These weren't just ordinary foods—they were divinely crafted, bursting with nutrients and healing properties to energize the body, sharpen the mind, and support spiritual connection.

Every fruit, seed, and herb was intentionally placed in Eden as part of God's perfect design for humanity's flourishing.

Over time, our diets have drifted far from this original plan. The processed foods and synthetic ingredients of today bear little resemblance to the pure, life-giving nourishment of Eden. Instead of vibrant health, we now face chronic illnesses, low energy, and a disconnection from God's natural rhythms. Yet, the foods God originally provided remain available to us. By rediscovering and embracing these superfoods, we can reclaim the vitality and spiritual alignment that are part of His divine design.

Modern science is beginning to validate what Scripture has proclaimed for centuries. Foods like figs, pomegranates, and herbs aren't just delicious—they're packed with compounds that heal the body and restore balance. Figs, for instance, are rich in fiber, which promotes gut health and regulates digestion, while their potassium content helps maintain healthy blood pressure. Similarly, pomegranates are brimming with antioxidants that repair damaged cells and combat inflammation, offering protection against chronic diseases like heart disease and diabetes. These are just two examples of the incredible power contained in the foods of Eden.

Here are some of the biblical superfoods you can incorporate into your life today:

BIBLICAL SUPERFOODS

- **Figs**: Support digestion, regulate blood pressure, and provide natural energy.
- **Pomegranates**: Fight inflammation and promote heart health with their rich antioxidant content.
- **Cumin**: Aids digestion, reduces inflammation, and adds a flavorful boost to meals.
- **Olives and Olive Oil**: Protect against heart disease, improve brain function, and reduce inflammation.
- **Honey**: A natural sweetener that boosts energy and supports the immune system.
- **Dates**: Packed with iron for energy and rich in fiber, dates are a perfect natural snack.
- **Grapes**: Contain resveratrol, which improves cardiovascular health and protects cells from damage.
- **Lentils**: A plant-based protein source rich in iron, fiber, and essential nutrients for sustained energy.
- **Barley**: Mentioned in the feeding of the 5,000, this grain is high in beta-glucans, which support heart health and digestion.

- **Mustard Seeds**: Known for their faith symbolism, these tiny seeds have anti-inflammatory properties and aid metabolism.

HOW TO INCORPORATE THESE SUPERFOODS INTO YOUR LIFE

The beauty of God's superfoods is that they're versatile and easy to incorporate into modern meals. Here are practical ways to use these foods daily:

1. **Breakfast Boost**: Start your day with a nutrient-packed breakfast by adding figs, dates, or pomegranate seeds to your oatmeal or yogurt. Top it with a drizzle of honey for natural sweetness and a handful of seeds like flax or chia to enhance digestion.
2. **Herbs in Cooking**: Use cumin, mustard seeds, and other herbs in soups, stews, and roasted vegetables. These small additions not only elevate flavor but also provide anti-inflammatory benefits. Mix a pinch of cumin with olive oil and lemon juice for a simple, health-boosting salad dressing.
3. **Healthy Snacks**: Swap processed snacks for portable options like dates, grapes, or a small bowl of mixed olives. These natural foods satisfy cravings while nourishing your body with essential vitamins and minerals.
4. **Hearty Meals**: Include lentils and barley in soups, salads, or as side dishes. Lentils provide plant-based protein and iron, making them a perfect alternative to meat, while barley's fiber supports digestion and sustained energy throughout the day.
5. **Sweet and Savory Enhancements**: Honey can be used not only as a natural sweetener in teas and baked goods but also as a glaze for roasted vegetables or meats. Its antimicrobial properties are an added health bonus.
6. **DIY Snacks**: Make a trail mix with roasted barley, mustard seeds, dried figs, and a touch of honey. This portable option combines the power of multiple superfoods in one bite, keeping you energized throughout the day.
7. **Olive Oil for Every Meal**: Use high-quality extra virgin olive oil for cooking, sautéing, or drizzling over meals. Its robust flavor enhances dishes while delivering heart-protective antioxidants.
8. **Beverage Boost**: Add a spoonful of honey to herbal teas infused with mint or thyme. This simple practice aligns with biblical traditions and provides a soothing, healthful drink.

<u>THE HEALING POWER OF FRUITS, HERBS, AND SEEDS</u>

The Bible is filled with examples of God using the natural world to provide healing. Fruits, herbs, and seeds are more than just nourishment—they are divinely designed tools for restoration and renewal. These foods were carefully chosen by God to address both the physical and spiritual needs of His people, and their inclusion in Scripture reveals profound truths about the connection between faith, health, and divine wisdom.

Consider the fig poultices used to heal King Hezekiah (Isaiah 38:21) or the bitter herbs consumed during Passover, which symbolized cleansing and purification. These instances are not just historical anecdotes; they represent a divine understanding of how food can act as medicine. When consumed with gratitude and intention, these natural gifts can support the body's ability to heal itself, reflecting God's care for His creation.

Biblical Wisdom and the Science of Healing

God's design for fruits, herbs, and seeds goes beyond sustenance; it anticipates modern discoveries about their medicinal properties. For example, herbs like mint and thyme were traditionally used for their soothing and purifying effects. Today, science confirms their antibacterial and anti-inflammatory benefits, proving the timelessness of God's wisdom.

Seeds, small but powerful, were given as symbols of life and regeneration. When Jesus compared faith to a mustard seed, He pointed to its potential to grow exponentially—just as the nutrients in seeds fuel vitality in the body. Flaxseeds, for instance, are now known to reduce inflammation and improve heart health, but they have been nourishing humanity since the dawn of agriculture. Each seed, herb, and fruit reflects God's foresight in equipping humanity with the tools to maintain health.

The Power of Intentional Eating

Eating these healing foods is more than a physical act—it's a spiritual practice that aligns us with God's original design. The Bible teaches us to approach food with gratitude and awareness, recognizing it as a gift from our Creator. Proverbs 3:8 reminds us that obedience to God's wisdom brings health to the body and nourishment to the bones. When we choose foods that honor His design, we also choose a path of obedience and trust.

The intentional use of fruits, herbs, and seeds can also serve as a reminder of the holistic nature of healing. These foods work synergistically with the body's natural processes, supporting digestion, reducing inflammation, and boosting immunity. In the same way, our spiritual health relies on aligning ourselves with God's rhythms—trusting Him for provision, resting in His care, and seeking Him in every aspect of our lives.

BIBLICAL OIL SECRETS THAT CHANGE EVERYTHING

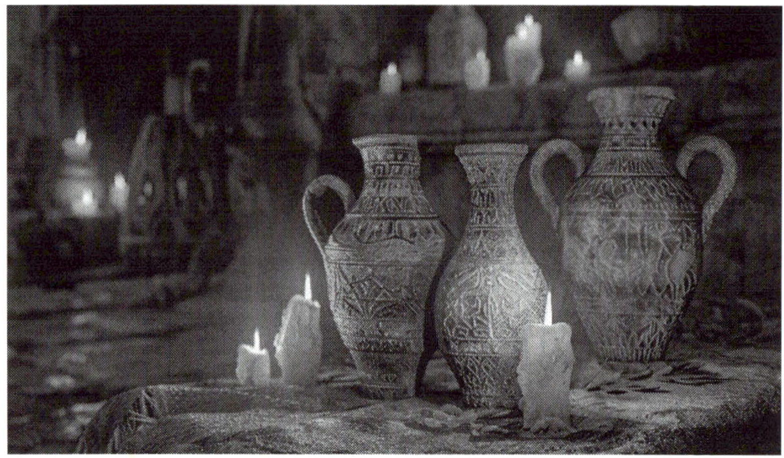

For centuries, oils have held a sacred place in Scripture, symbolizing anointing, healing, and divine blessing. From the olive oil that fueled the lamps in the Tabernacle to the myrrh and frankincense offered to the infant Jesus, oils were more than practical—they were spiritual tools imbued with profound significance. These ancient oils were revered not only for their symbolic power but also for their transformative physical properties. They healed wounds, purified bodies, and brought strength and vitality to those who used them.

Modern science now validates what Scripture has proclaimed for millennia: oils like olive, myrrh, and frankincense possess extraordinary health benefits. Rich in antioxidants, anti-inflammatory compounds, and healing properties, these oils have the power to transform health and wellness. In this chapter, we'll uncover the biblical secrets of these sacred oils, exploring their significance in God's Word and their incredible potential to restore and rejuvenate in today's world.

OLIVE OIL: THE SACRED ELIXIR OF THE BIBLE

Few substances are as deeply intertwined with biblical history and tradition as olive oil. It was the oil used to anoint kings, priests, and prophets, signifying divine favor and purpose. Olive oil illuminated the lamps of the Tabernacle and played a central role in offerings and sacred rituals (Exodus 27:20). Beyond its spiritual significance, olive oil was also a cornerstone of daily life in biblical times—valued for its ability to heal, nourish, and sustain.

Modern research has revealed what the ancient world instinctively knew: olive oil is a gift to the body. Rich in monounsaturated fats, it protects the heart by lowering bad cholesterol (LDL) while boosting good cholesterol (HDL). Olive oil is also packed with polyphenols, powerful antioxidants that combat inflammation and oxidative stress—two key drivers of chronic illness. Its anti-inflammatory properties are so potent that they mimic the effects of ibuprofen, reducing pain and promoting overall health.

How to Use Olive Oil Today

1. **Cooking and Drizzling**: Use extra virgin olive oil as your go-to fat for cooking, sautéing, or drizzling over vegetables and salads. Its high-quality fats and antioxidants make it an ideal choice for heart health.
2. **Skin Care**: Apply olive oil directly to dry skin or use it as a base for homemade moisturizers. Its natural antioxidants and vitamin E content promote hydration and healing.
3. **Traditional Remedies**: Combine olive oil with a touch of honey and lemon for a soothing remedy for sore throats or indigestion, a practice rooted in ancient traditions.

The biblical reverence for olive oil wasn't just spiritual; it reflected God's wisdom in providing humanity with a substance that sustains the body and symbolizes His anointing power. Incorporating olive oil into your life today honors this tradition while embracing its incredible health benefits.

MYRRH AND FRANKINCENSE: ANCIENT HEALING WONDERS

In the Bible, myrrh and frankincense are not mere commodities; they are treasures with profound spiritual and practical significance. Offered as gifts to the infant Jesus (Matthew 2:11), these aromatic resins symbolized royalty, divinity, and the ultimate act of worship. Myrrh was used for purification, embalming, and as a key ingredient in anointing oils, while frankincense was central to offerings and incense, representing prayers rising to heaven (Exodus 30:34).

Beyond their sacred symbolism, myrrh and frankincense hold extraordinary healing properties. Myrrh is a powerful antiseptic and anti-inflammatory agent, used historically to treat wounds, infections, and respiratory conditions. Frankincense, known for its calming and uplifting aroma, supports immune health, reduces inflammation, and even aids in cellular regeneration. Together, these oils serve as potent reminders of the connection between spiritual worship and physical healing.

How to Use Myrrh and Frankincense Today

1. **Aromatherapy**: Diffuse frankincense in your home to promote relaxation, mental clarity, and a prayerful atmosphere.
2. **Skin Healing**: Dilute myrrh with a carrier oil (like olive or coconut oil) and apply it to wounds, cuts, or dry skin for its antibacterial and healing properties.
3. **Immune Support**: Add a few drops of frankincense oil to a warm bath or mix it with a carrier oil for a soothing massage to support the immune system and reduce stress.

These ancient oils bridge the gap between the physical and spiritual, reminding us that God's provision for health is holistic. By incorporating myrrh and frankincense into your life, you connect with biblical traditions while benefiting from their timeless healing power.

THE SCIENCE BEHIND SCRIPTURE'S HEALING OILS

Modern science has uncovered the extraordinary properties of the oils revered in Scripture, confirming their role as powerful natural remedies. Olive oil, a staple in biblical times, is now celebrated for its heart-protective properties. Research shows that its high levels of monounsaturated fats, particularly oleic acid, help lower bad cholesterol (LDL) and raise good cholesterol (HDL). In addition, the polyphenols in olive oil act as potent antioxidants, reducing inflammation and oxidative stress—both major contributors to heart disease and chronic illness. A 2013 study published in *The New England Journal of Medicine* even demonstrated that a Mediterranean diet rich in olive oil significantly reduced the risk of cardiovascular events like strokes and heart attacks.

Frankincense, often used in biblical worship and rituals, is now recognized for its therapeutic impact on the immune and nervous systems. Studies have shown that frankincense contains boswellic acids, which have strong anti-inflammatory and anti-cancer properties. Research published in *Cancer Research* highlights its ability to inhibit the growth of cancer cells, particularly in conditions such as leukemia and breast cancer. Additionally, frankincense has been shown to alleviate symptoms of anxiety and depression by interacting with receptors in the brain, reducing cortisol levels, and promoting relaxation. These findings confirm that the biblical use of frankincense as an agent of purification and healing was not merely symbolic—it was profoundly functional.

Myrrh, another oil with deep biblical significance, is valued today for its antimicrobial and anti-inflammatory properties. A 2012 study in *Evidence-Based Complementary and Alternative Medicine* revealed that myrrh extracts effectively inhibit the growth of harmful bacteria and fungi, making it a powerful natural alternative to synthetic antibiotics. Additionally, myrrh's active compounds have been shown to reduce inflammation, aiding in the treatment of conditions such as arthritis and digestive issues. Its use in embalming and purification rituals in

Scripture aligns with its proven ability to preserve and protect organic matter—a testament to the wisdom embedded in biblical practices.

Even the application of these oils as inhalants or topical remedies reveals insights into their physiological benefits. Frankincense, when diffused, releases aromatic compounds that stimulate the limbic system in the brain, influencing emotions, memory, and focus. Myrrh, applied to wounds, accelerates healing through its antiseptic properties. Olive oil, used as a carrier oil, enhances the absorption of active ingredients in other medicinal oils while nourishing and protecting the skin. The scientific validation of these properties highlights how biblical oils address modern health challenges, bridging the gap between ancient wisdom and contemporary science.

Why Biblical Oils Still Matter

- **They bridge the sacred and the physical**: Oils like myrrh and frankincense remind us that healing isn't purely mechanical. They engage the senses, helping us reconnect with God as we restore our bodies.
- **They're backed by modern science**: From olive oil's heart-protective properties to frankincense's ability to calm the nervous system, these oils stand the test of time.
- **They're natural solutions**: At a time when synthetic treatments dominate, these oils offer a cleaner, simpler way to support wellness.

DIY SACRED OIL REMEDIES FOR HOME AND BODY

The oils referenced in Scripture aren't just powerful; they're versatile. With a little creativity, you can use them to create effective, natural remedies for everyday needs—right in your own home. From skincare to stress relief, these DIY recipes draw on ancient wisdom while addressing modern challenges, offering a simple yet profound way to embrace the healing properties of biblical oils.

1. Calming Frankincense Diffuser Blend
Harness the calming power of frankincense with this easy diffuser blend. Perfect for moments of prayer, meditation, or relaxation, this aromatic recipe promotes emotional balance and reduces stress.

- **Ingredients**: 4 drops frankincense oil, 2 drops lavender oil, 2 drops bergamot oil, and water (as required by your diffuser).
- **Instructions**: Add the oils and water to your diffuser and let the soothing aroma fill your space. This blend not only calms the mind but also uplifts the spirit, creating an atmosphere of peace and focus.

2. Healing Myrrh Wound Salve

Inspired by myrrh's use in biblical healing, this salve can cleanse and protect minor wounds or irritated skin.

- **Ingredients**: 1 tablespoon coconut oil, 1 tablespoon beeswax, 5 drops myrrh oil, 3 drops tea tree oil.
- **Instructions**: Melt the coconut oil and beeswax together in a double boiler. Remove from heat and stir in the oils. Pour the mixture into a small container and allow it to cool and solidify. Apply a small amount to wounds or cuts to support healing.

3. Luxurious Olive Oil Hair Treatment

Olive oil's nourishing properties make it a perfect remedy for dry or damaged hair. This simple treatment restores shine and moisture while strengthening your locks.

- **Ingredients**: 2 tablespoons extra virgin olive oil and 1 tablespoon honey.
- **Instructions**: Mix the olive oil and honey in a small bowl. Apply the mixture to clean, damp hair, focusing on the ends. Leave it on for 20-30 minutes, then rinse thoroughly with warm water and shampoo. Use weekly for best results.

4. Revitalizing Anointing Oil for Daily Use

Create your own anointing oil to incorporate into your daily routine for spiritual and physical renewal. This blend is inspired by the sacred oils of Scripture and can be used for prayer, massage, or relaxation.

- **Ingredients**: 1/4 cup olive oil, 5 drops frankincense oil, 3 drops myrrh oil, and 2 drops cinnamon oil.
- **Instructions**: Combine the ingredients in a small glass bottle. Shake gently before each use. Apply a small amount to your wrists or neck during prayer or reflection as a way to connect with the sacred traditions of anointing.

5. Soothing Foot Bath with Biblical Oils

Relax tired feet and promote circulation with a warm foot bath infused with the healing properties of myrrh and olive oil.

- **Ingredients**: 2 tablespoons olive oil, 3 drops myrrh oil, 1/2 cup Epsom salt, and warm water.
- **Instructions**: Dissolve the Epsom salt in a basin of warm water, then add the oils. Soak your feet for 15-20 minutes. This bath not only soothes aches but also softens skin and enhances relaxation.

6. Cedarwood Sleep-Enhancing Pillow Spray

Cedarwood, often associated with purity and sanctuary in the Bible, promotes deep relaxation and restful sleep.

- **Ingredients**: 1/2 cup distilled water, 10 drops cedarwood essential oil, 5 drops lavender oil.
- **Instructions**: Combine the ingredients in a spray bottle and shake well. Lightly mist your pillow before bedtime to create a calming and sleep-friendly environment.

7. Spikenard Relaxation Massage Oil

Spikenard, used to anoint Jesus (John 12:3), has calming and grounding properties, making it ideal for relaxation and stress relief.

- **Ingredients**: 2 tablespoons almond oil, 6 drops spikenard essential oil, 3 drops bergamot oil.
- **Instructions**: Mix the oils and use for a gentle, soothing massage to reduce tension and promote relaxation.

8. Cassia Energizing Body Oil

Known as a key ingredient in the holy anointing oil (Exodus 30:22-25), cassia has a warm, uplifting aroma that stimulates energy and circulation.

- **Ingredients**: 2 tablespoons olive oil, 5 drops cassia essential oil, 3 drops orange essential oil.
- **Instructions**: Blend the oils in a small bottle. Apply to your arms and legs in the morning to invigorate your body and boost circulation.

9. Hyssop Cleansing Steam for Respiratory Support

Hyssop, mentioned in Psalm 51:7 as a purifier, is ideal for supporting respiratory health.

- **Ingredients**: 3 drops hyssop essential oil, 1 drop peppermint essential oil, 1 quart steaming water.
- **Instructions**: Add the oils to a bowl of steaming water. Drape a towel over your head and inhale deeply for 5–10 minutes. This steam clears sinuses and supports lung health.

10. Cinnamon and Cassia Immune-Boosting Chest Rub

Cinnamon and cassia, often paired in Scripture, are known for their warming and antimicrobial properties. This chest rub soothes and supports immunity during cold seasons.

- **Ingredients**: 2 tablespoons coconut oil, 3 drops cassia essential oil, 2 drops cinnamon essential oil, 1 drop eucalyptus oil.
- **Instructions**: Mix the ingredients in a small jar. Rub a small amount onto your chest to ease congestion and support immune health.

GOD'S SECRET WEAPON FOR TOTAL RENEWAL

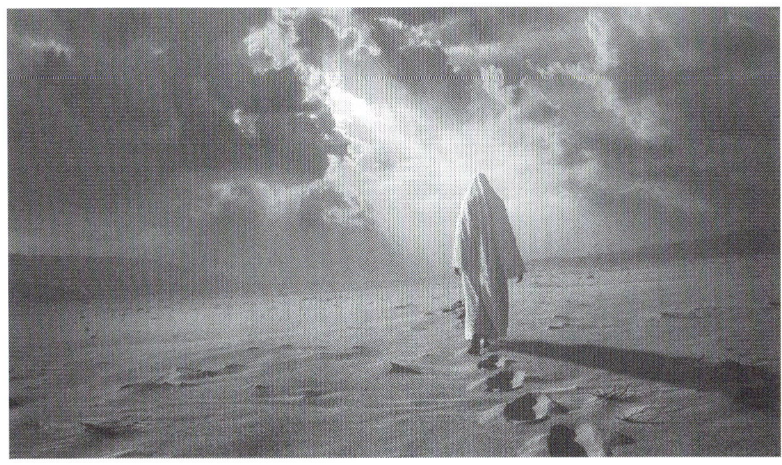

In the Bible, one practice stands out as a divine strategy for physical and spiritual renewal: fasting. This sacred discipline, commanded and modeled throughout Scripture, is far more than just abstaining from food. It's a holistic reset—a way to purify the body, sharpen the mind, and draw closer to God. From Moses on Mount Sinai to Jesus in the wilderness, fasting has always been a powerful tool for transformation and alignment with God's will.

The physical benefits of fasting are just as profound as the spiritual ones. Modern science now affirms what the Bible has always taught: fasting activates the body's natural ability to heal and regenerate. It triggers autophagy, a process where cells clean themselves of damaged components, leading to improved energy, mental clarity, and even longevity. By giving the digestive system a rest, fasting allows the body to focus on repair and renewal, making it a practice that rejuvenates from the inside out.

But fasting isn't just about health; it's about surrender. In a world driven by consumption, fasting reminds us that we are sustained by more than food—it is God who provides, heals, and restores. This chapter will uncover the biblical significance of fasting, explore its extraordinary physical and spiritual benefits, and guide you on how to begin this transformative practice. Whether you're seeking healing, clarity, or a deeper connection with God, fasting is the secret weapon that unlocks renewal in every part of your life.

FASTING: GOD'S COMMAND FOR SPIRITUAL STRENGTH

Fasting is not just an act of self-denial—it is a sacred process that works on two fronts: it purifies the body and fortifies the soul. The wisdom of fasting lies in its ability to strip away what is unnecessary, allowing both the physical and spiritual to renew and regenerate. This is not a mere health trend or spiritual exercise; it is a divine practice, embedded in God's design for human flourishing.

Physically, fasting is a biological masterpiece of renewal. During a fast, the body enters a state of autophagy, a term derived from Greek meaning "self-eating." This process is nothing short of miraculous: the body begins to identify and eliminate damaged cells, toxins, and unnecessary debris, leaving a cleaner, more efficient system. In essence, fasting triggers the body's God-given ability to heal itself. This cleansing doesn't just benefit the body's internal systems—it recharges energy, sharpens the mind, and reduces inflammation, which is a root cause of many chronic diseases. It's as though fasting presses the reset button on your physical health, a practice that science has only recently begun to understand but that Scripture has long affirmed.

Spiritually, fasting is an act of submission and trust. It is a declaration that our reliance on God outweighs our dependence on physical sustenance. By choosing to abstain from food, we symbolically and literally empty ourselves, making room for God to fill the void. This alignment of physical hunger with spiritual hunger creates a heightened awareness of God's presence. Joel 2:12 calls believers to "return to me with all your heart, with fasting." This act of humility purifies not just the body, but also the heart, breaking down pride and distractions to refocus on God's grace and provision.

The beauty of fasting lies in how it unites these two processes: physical cleansing and spiritual strengthening. It's not just about what you're giving up—it's about what you're gaining. As the body sheds toxins, the spirit sheds burdens. As physical cravings subside, spiritual clarity emerges. Fasting is a divine rhythm that reminds us of our Creator's wisdom, a practice that heals and strengthens in tandem.

How Fasting Purifies and Strengthens

- **Heightened Spiritual Focus**: Fasting clears distractions, allowing deeper connection and alignment with God's will.
- **Energy Realignment**: Without the constant need for digestion, the body redirects energy toward healing and regeneration, mirroring the spiritual redirection of focus to God.

- **Humility and Dependence**: Fasting fosters reliance on God's provision, strengthening faith and trust in His sustenance.

Fasting is more than the sum of its parts—it is a divinely orchestrated pathway to restoration. Each hunger pang becomes a reminder of God's provision; each physical renewal mirrors the deeper renewal of the spirit. This is not deprivation—it is empowerment, a reminder that both body and soul are intricately connected in God's plan for renewal and strength.

THE MIRACULOUS HEALTH BENEFITS OF BIBLICAL FASTING

Fasting is far more than a spiritual discipline—it is a profound biological process that unlocks the body's God-designed ability to heal and rejuvenate itself. Modern science has begun to uncover what the Bible has long affirmed: fasting is a catalyst for physical restoration, mental clarity, and even extended longevity. These health benefits are not incidental; they are integral to God's plan for renewal, as fasting provides a reset for both body and mind.

Autophagy: The Body's Self-Cleaning Mechanism

At the heart of fasting's physical benefits is a process called autophagy, a word derived from Greek meaning "self-eating." When the body enters a fasting state, it begins to clean house. Damaged cells, toxic proteins, and worn-out components are broken down and recycled for energy or repair. This miraculous process, discovered by scientists only recently, has been linked to reduced inflammation, improved immune function, and protection against neurodegenerative diseases like Alzheimer's. Autophagy is like God's built-in maintenance system, activated when we give the body time to rest from constant digestion. It's no surprise that this cellular cleansing aligns so perfectly with the biblical concept of fasting as purification.

Improved Focus and Mental Clarity

One of the most immediate benefits of fasting is heightened mental clarity. During fasting, the body shifts from burning glucose to burning ketones—a more efficient fuel source for the brain. This metabolic shift often leads to sharper focus, quicker decision-making, and a sense of heightened awareness. It's as though fasting sweeps away the mental fog, clearing space for deeper reflection and connection. This mental clarity may explain why fasting is so often paired with prayer in Scripture; it helps remove distractions, enabling believers to hear God's voice more clearly.

Longevity: Extending Life Through Renewal

Fasting has also been shown to slow the aging process and extend life. Studies on intermittent fasting and caloric restriction reveal that periodic fasting reduces oxidative stress, a major contributor to cellular aging. By promoting autophagy and reducing chronic inflammation, fasting protects cells from the damage that accelerates aging. Cultures with fasting traditions, such as those in the Mediterranean region, often experience longer lifespans and better overall health. The biblical command to fast isn't just a spiritual exercise—it's a tool for maintaining the vitality needed to fulfill God's purpose throughout a long and fruitful life.

Key Health Benefits of Fasting

- **Cellular Repair**: Activates autophagy, removing damaged cells and toxins.
- **Neuroprotection**: Supports brain health and reduces the risk of diseases like Alzheimer's.
- **Mental Clarity**: Sharpens focus and enhances cognitive performance.
- **Reduced Inflammation**: Lowers inflammation throughout the body, decreasing the risk of chronic illness.
- **Longevity**: Slows the aging process and promotes a longer, healthier life.

Fasting is a gift from God that brings the body into alignment with His rhythms of restoration. By embracing this practice, we step into a cycle of renewal that touches every aspect of our being—physical, mental, and spiritual.

A STEP-BY-STEP GUIDE TO YOUR FIRST FAST

Embarking on a biblical fast may feel daunting, but it's a practice rooted in simplicity and intention. The key to success is to start small and approach the process with both physical preparation and spiritual focus. Whether your goal is to deepen your faith, seek clarity, or improve your health, this guide will walk you through the steps of your first fast, making it an achievable and transformative experience.

1. Choose Your Fast Type
Decide what kind of fast you will undertake. Options include:

- **Complete Fast**: Abstaining from all food and consuming only water.
- **Partial Fast**: Skipping one or two meals a day or abstaining from certain food groups (like Daniel's fast of vegetables and water in Daniel 1:12).
- **Intermittent Fast**: Limiting eating to a specific window of time each day (e.g., 16 hours fasting, 8 hours eating).

2. Set Your Intentions
Define the purpose of your fast. Are you seeking spiritual guidance, healing, or

focus? Write down your intentions and commit to pairing your fast with prayer or Scripture meditation to stay spiritually anchored.

3. Prepare Your Body
Ease into your fast by gradually reducing portion sizes and cutting out processed foods a few days beforehand. Stay hydrated and avoid indulging in heavy meals right before your fast begins.

4. Select a Start and End Time
Choose a specific start and end time for your fast. Knowing the duration helps you stay focused and committed. For beginners, a short 12- to 24-hour fast is a manageable starting point.

5. Stay Hydrated
Drink plenty of water throughout your fast to avoid dehydration and help your body cleanse itself more effectively. If your fast permits, herbal teas can be included as well.

6. Engage in Prayer and Reflection
Use the time you would normally spend eating to pray, read Scripture, or reflect. Fasting is not just about abstaining from food; it's about seeking God and aligning with His will.

7. Break Your Fast Wisely
When your fast ends, break it gently with light, nourishing foods like fruits, vegetables, or broths. Avoid heavy or processed meals, as your digestive system will need time to readjust.

8. Reflect on Your Experience
After your fast, take time to reflect on what you learned—both physically and spiritually. Write down any insights, answers to prayer, or lessons God revealed during the process.

This step-by-step approach makes fasting approachable while keeping its sacred purpose front and center. With preparation and intention, your first fast can become a powerful act of renewal and transformation.

MOVE LIKE THE PROPHETS AND TRANSFORM YOUR BODY

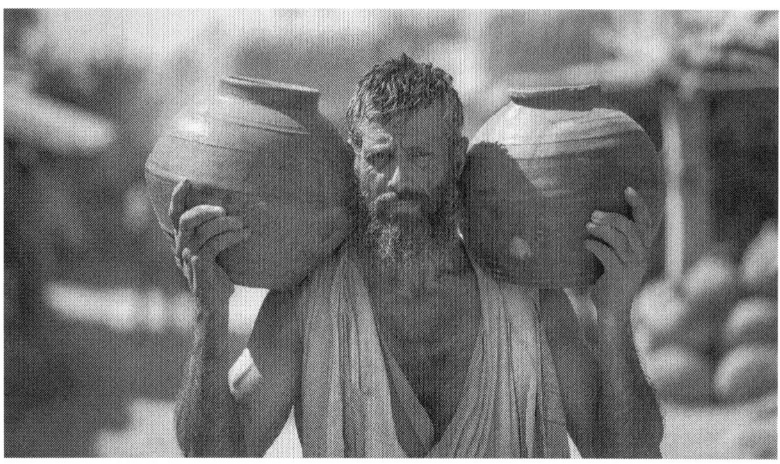

What if the key to vibrant health wasn't hidden in a gym or a fitness app, but in the very pages of Scripture? The Bible may not mention treadmills or spin classes, but it reveals a lifestyle of movement that built resilience, strength, and endurance. From shepherds roaming rugged hills to carpenters shaping wood by hand, the physical activities of biblical figures were purposeful, intense, and deeply connected to God's creation. Their lives demanded a kind of functional fitness that modern routines often overlook—a fitness that wasn't about aesthetics, but about living fully and faithfully.

Today, we live in a world of convenience, where movement has been replaced by screens and chairs, and health is undermined by inactivity. Yet the Bible offers a countercultural solution: a return to the purposeful, intentional movement of the prophets and disciples. This chapter will uncover the hidden wisdom in biblical forms of labor and activity, exploring how simple, meaningful movements can transform your health, restore your energy, and connect you to a rhythm of life that honors both your body and your Creator. Get ready to rethink how you move and why it matters.

BIBLICAL LABOR: THE SECRET TO RESILIENT STRENGTH

The work of biblical times wasn't for the faint of heart. It was raw, physical, and often grueling—but it forged strength, both of body and spirit. Shepherds like David, builders like Noah, and laborers in the fields weren't just surviving; they were thriving in a way that modern, sedentary lifestyles often fail to replicate. These tasks demanded endurance, power, and focus, shaping resilient individuals whose physical work mirrored their spiritual devotion.

Examples of Biblical Labor That Built Strength

- **Shepherding**: Constant movement, navigating rocky terrains, and defending flocks from predators like lions and bears built core stability, reflexes, and endurance.
- **Building**: Tasks like lifting timber and stone, cutting materials, and assembling massive structures like the Ark or the Temple required immense physical strength and stamina.
- **Threshing and Grinding Grain**: Repeated, labor-intensive motions such as separating wheat from chaff and grinding it into flour kept arms and shoulders strong.
- **Fishing**: The act of casting nets into the sea and hauling them back, often filled with heavy fish, worked the entire body, particularly the arms, back, and core.

These were not isolated moments of exertion; they were the fabric of daily life. Shepherding, for example, required navigating hills, chasing wandering sheep, and standing watch through the night. It was a constant test of endurance and adaptability, especially for figures like David, who faced physical challenges that prepared him for future battles. Building, too, was monumental in scale. Consider Noah's Ark: it wasn't a weekend project but decades of relentless cutting, hauling, and constructing a massive vessel—an act of obedience that demanded unwavering focus and strength.

But these tasks were more than physical; they were deeply purposeful. Shepherds weren't just tending sheep—they were protecting vital resources for their families and communities. Builders weren't just assembling structures—they were fulfilling divine commands, creating spaces for worship and protection. The intentionality behind these acts gave every motion meaning, transforming what might seem like simple labor into acts of faith and devotion.

How Biblical Labor Strengthened the Body

- **Total-Body Conditioning**: Activities like shepherding and fishing required endurance, balance, and strength, engaging multiple muscle groups simultaneously.
- **Stamina Building**: Daily labor, such as threshing or building, demanded sustained effort, building cardiovascular endurance over time.

- **Functional Movement**: These activities mimicked real-world challenges, such as carrying heavy loads or navigating rough terrain, resulting in practical, usable strength.
- **Resilience**: The repetitive nature of these tasks cultivated mental toughness and physical durability, traits essential for thriving in challenging environments.

Biblical labor wasn't just work—it was worship in motion, a rhythm of life that strengthened the body while anchoring the spirit to God's greater purpose.

MODERN WORKOUTS INSPIRED BY THE PROPHETS' MOVEMENTS

The physical tasks performed by prophets, shepherds, and builders in biblical times weren't just work—they were full-body workouts that built strength, stamina, and resilience. Today, we can draw inspiration from these purposeful movements to create modern routines that are both practical and meaningful. These exercises aren't about logging hours at the gym; they're about reconnecting with the kinds of functional movements God designed our bodies to perform. By mimicking the natural labor of biblical figures, we can cultivate strength that serves us in daily life while fostering a deeper sense of purpose.

Biblical-Inspired Exercises for Modern Routines

- **Walking**: Emulate the long journeys of Jesus and the prophets by taking extended walks outdoors. Walking strengthens endurance, improves cardiovascular health, and fosters mindfulness.
- **Rowing Motions**: Inspired by fishermen casting and pulling nets, use resistance bands or rowing machines to replicate the pulling actions that strengthen the arms, shoulders, and back.
- **Ground Work**: Mimic agricultural tasks like threshing grain by performing dynamic movements such as twisting woodchoppers or kettlebell swings, which target the core and improve mobility.
- **Step-Ups**: Mimic the terrain-navigation of shepherds by stepping up onto a sturdy surface like a bench or a step. This movement strengthens the legs, glutes, and core while improving balance.
- **Farmer's Carry**: Carry heavy objects like buckets of water in each hand, similar to tasks in biblical agriculture. This builds grip strength, core stability, and endurance.
- **Push-Pulls**: Combine pushing and pulling motions with resistance bands to replicate the strength required for tasks like opening gates or hauling loads. This targets upper body and core strength.

- **Sledgehammer Swings**: Using a weighted hammer or similar tool, mimic the movements of striking or breaking materials during construction. This full-body exercise improves power and coordination.
- **Overhead Carries**: Carry a heavy object, such as a weight or backpack, overhead while walking. This strengthens the shoulders, core, and stability, mimicking the act of carrying tools or supplies for building.
- **Box Pulls**: Drag a heavy box or sled across the floor to replicate the pulling motions used in tasks like fishing nets or moving stones. This targets the legs, arms, and back.
- **Log or Stone Lifts**: Use a weighted object like a sandbag to simulate lifting logs or stones as builders and laborers did. This movement improves strength and coordination.
- **Step-Back Lunges**: Perform lunges by stepping backward instead of forward, building lower body strength and balance. This reflects movements like bending and stepping during farming or construction.
- **Bear Crawls**: Move on all fours, mimicking the functional strength and coordination required for tasks like threshing grain or gathering materials from the ground.

These exercises aren't just about physical fitness; they align with how our bodies were meant to move—functionally and intentionally. For example, walking isn't just cardio; it's an opportunity to reflect on biblical journeys and connect with God through prayer. Weighted carries not only build strength but also improve balance and coordination, echoing the focus and discipline of shepherds protecting their flocks. Every movement has a purpose, and when you approach exercise this way, it transcends physical fitness to become a spiritual practice.

By grounding your workouts in biblical inspiration, you're also cultivating resilience. Think of the repetitive labor of threshing or building—tasks that required strength over time, not in short bursts. These movements build endurance and perseverance, qualities essential for both physical and spiritual growth. You're not just lifting weights; you're preparing your body and mind for the challenges of daily life, just as the prophets and disciples did.

How to Start Incorporating Biblical Movements

1. Begin each day with a 20-30 minute walk, reflecting on Scripture or praying as you move.
2. Practice simple weighted carries, holding bags or weights while walking around your home or yard.
3. Perform lifting motions like squats and presses 2-3 times a week to build functional strength.
4. Incorporate resistance band rows or kettlebell swings into your routine to simulate biblical pulling and threshing motions.

5. Make movement a daily habit, not a chore—view each exercise as a way to honor the body God gave you.
6. Incorporate Everyday Items: Use household items like jugs of water, grocery bags, or furniture to perform resistance and carrying exercises, mirroring the practicality of biblical labor.
7. Make It a Family Activity: Engage your family or friends in group walks or shared tasks like gardening to echo the communal aspects of labor in Scripture.
8. Add Movement to Prayer Time: Combine spiritual practices with physical activity by praying or meditating while performing repetitive movements like walking or rowing.
9. Create a Functional Circuit: Design a workout circuit with 5-6 biblical-inspired movements (e.g., walking, lifting, and carrying) for a 20-minute session that mimics the variety of tasks in a day's labor.
10. Tie Movements to Scripture: Choose a verse or biblical story tied to each exercise to inspire your workout. For example, reflect on David's strength as a shepherd while performing weighted carries.

These routines aren't about perfection or performance. They're about embodying the wisdom of Scripture in every step, lift, and pull, transforming ordinary exercise into an extraordinary connection to the Creator.

THE BIBLICAL MOVEMENT CHALLENGE YOU CAN START TODAY

Transforming your body and spirit doesn't require a gym membership or a drastic overhaul of your life—it starts with a simple commitment. The Biblical Movement Challenge is designed to reconnect you with the purposeful, strength-building activities of Scripture. Over the next seven days, you'll engage in movements inspired by shepherds, builders, and disciples, cultivating resilience and mindfulness. This isn't just a physical exercise; it's a spiritual journey, aligning your daily actions with the rhythms of God's creation.

The 7-Day Biblical Movement Challenge

1. **Day 1: Walk with Purpose**
    Take a 20-minute walk outdoors, reflecting on a Scripture passage like Psalm 23:1-3. Focus on moving intentionally, just as biblical figures walked miles each day.
2. **Day 2: Weighted Carry**
    Carry a weighted object (such as a backpack or a bucket) for 5 minutes, mimicking the strength of shepherds and builders. Rest and repeat for three rounds.
3. **Day 3: Lifting Practice**
    Perform 10 squats and 10 overhead lifts with a heavy object, such as a

bag of rice or a small crate. Complete three rounds to build functional strength.
4.   **Day 4: Restorative Movement**
Spend 15 minutes stretching or practicing gentle yoga-inspired poses while meditating on Matthew 11:28-30. Allow your body to recover and reflect on God's gift of rest.
5.   **Day 5: Rowing or Pulling Motion**
Use resistance bands, a rowing machine, or mimic pulling motions to strengthen your back, shoulders, and arms. Aim for 15 minutes of steady effort.
6.   **Day 6: Long Walk**
Extend your walking time to 30 minutes. Choose a route that challenges you with hills or uneven terrain, reflecting on the endurance of Jesus and His disciples.
7.   **Day 7: Reflection and Gratitude**
Combine light movement (such as a 10-minute walk) with prayer, thanking God for your body and the strength He provides. Reflect on the week's progress and set intentions for continued practice.

This challenge is more than a workout—it's a way to ground yourself in purpose. Each movement is inspired by Scripture, reminding you of the connection between physical strength and spiritual obedience. As you progress, you'll discover that these simple activities have profound effects on your body, mind, and faith.

Every step you take, every lift you make, mirrors the purposeful lives of biblical figures. This is not just a routine—it's a way to honor God's creation and design. By starting today, you're stepping into a rhythm of renewal, building the resilience to thrive physically and spiritually.

GOD'S ETERNAL YOUTH FORMULA HIDDEN FOR AGES

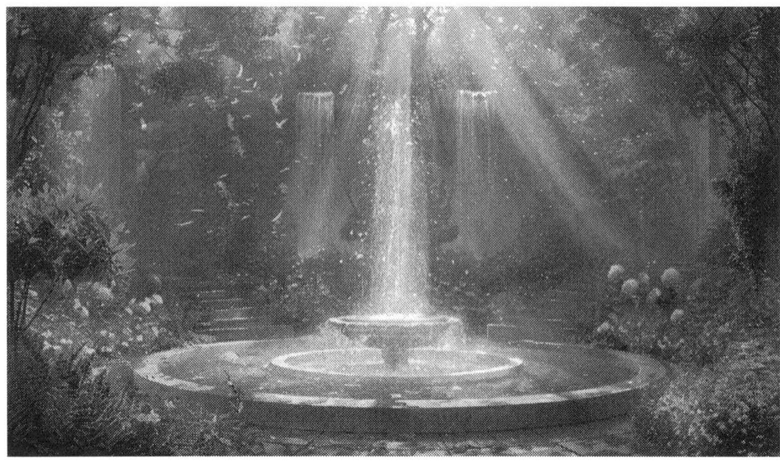

What if the secret to vitality and longevity wasn't found in modern medicine but in the timeless wisdom of Scripture? The Bible is filled with stories of extraordinary lifespans—Methuselah living 969 years, Abraham fathering a child at 100, and Sarah laughing at the prospect of renewed strength in her old age. These weren't mythical exaggerations; they were the result of living in harmony with God's design. This chapter unveils the biblical principles of longevity, exploring how faith, gratitude, and obedience to God's rhythms can unlock vitality that defies the years. Hidden in plain sight, the formula for eternal youth isn't a mystery—it's a divine gift, waiting for you to rediscover it.

THE BIBLE'S LONGEVITY SECRETS FINALLY UNCOVERED

The Bible is filled with accounts of people living lives that far exceeded modern expectations. Figures like Methuselah, Noah, and Adam didn't just survive—they thrived, living for centuries in harmony with God's design. These lifespans weren't random; they were the result of habits, environments, and faith practices deeply rooted in obedience to God. Their stories invite us to uncover the principles that contributed to their longevity and explore how we can integrate those practices into our lives today.

Biblical Figures and Their Lifespans

- **Methuselah**: 969 years (Genesis 5:27)
- **Adam**: 930 years (Genesis 5:5)
- **Noah**: 950 years (Genesis 9:29)
- **Seth**: 912 years (Genesis 5:8)
- **Enosh**: 905 years (Genesis 5:11)
- **Kenan**: 910 years (Genesis 5:14)
- **Mahalalel**: 895 years (Genesis 5:17)
- **Jared**: 962 years (Genesis 5:20)
- **Lamech (Noah's father)**: 777 years (Genesis 5:31)
- **Abraham**: 175 years (Genesis 25:7)
- **Sarah**: 127 years (Genesis 23:1)

These figures lived lives of astonishing length, but their longevity wasn't just a biological anomaly—it was deeply connected to how they lived.

Harmony with Creation

Many of these biblical figures lived in close connection to the natural world, free from the environmental toxins and processed foods that dominate modern life. Their diets consisted of untainted, God-given foods like fruits, grains, and seed-bearing plants, as described in Genesis 1:29. Their daily lives involved physical labor—tending fields, shepherding flocks, and building—that kept their bodies active and resilient. This alignment with creation wasn't just practical; it reflected an intentional harmony with God's design.

Faith and Obedience

A common thread among these figures is their unwavering faith in and obedience to God. Noah, for instance, trusted God's instructions to build the Ark, despite the ridicule and challenges he faced (Genesis 6:22). This obedience wasn't passive—it was an active choice that shaped their lives and cultivated a sense of purpose. Faith and obedience are repeatedly linked to health and longevity in Scripture, as in Deuteronomy 5:33: "Walk in obedience to all that the Lord your God has commanded you, so that you may live long and prosper."

Rest and Renewal

The Bible emphasizes the importance of rest, and these long-lived figures likely observed rhythms of work and Sabbath that allowed their bodies and spirits to renew. The practice of resting on the seventh day, established by God in Genesis 2:2-3, wasn't just spiritual—it was restorative. Modern science affirms that regular rest reduces stress, supports immune function, and promotes longevity, underscoring the wisdom of this ancient practice.

Gratitude and Purpose

Living with gratitude and a clear sense of purpose was another hallmark of these biblical figures. Abraham's journey was filled with faith-driven purpose as he followed God's promise to make him the father of nations (Genesis 12:1-3). This alignment with a greater mission gave their lives meaning, reducing the emotional and psychological burdens that can undermine health. Gratitude and purpose are known to improve mental health, lower stress, and extend life, showing a tangible connection between faith and longevity.

Generational Impact

These long-lived figures often saw their lifespans as opportunities to influence multiple generations. Methuselah, for example, would have witnessed the lives of many descendants, fostering a legacy of wisdom and faith. This generational connection deepened their sense of community and responsibility, traits that modern studies associate with better health and longer lifespans.

The longevity of these biblical figures wasn't just a gift—it was a reflection of their lifestyles, faith, and alignment with God's design. Their stories are an invitation to rediscover the rhythms and principles that can restore vitality and purpose in our own lives.

HOW FAITH AND GRATITUDE ADD YEARS TO YOUR LIFE

Gratitude is not merely a modern wellness trend; it's a divine directive deeply embedded in scripture. When Paul urged the Thessalonians to "give thanks in all circumstances" (1 Thessalonians 5:18), he wasn't offering empty platitudes. Gratitude in biblical times wasn't circumstantial—it was a discipline of the soul. From David's psalms of thanksgiving to Jesus giving thanks before breaking bread, gratitude threads through scripture as a powerful spiritual practice.

Consider Job. His steadfast gratitude amid loss exemplifies the profound spiritual and physical resilience that comes from trusting God. Gratitude in the Bible often aligns with healing and restoration. Naaman, the Syrian commander, was healed of leprosy after following Elisha's instructions and expressing humble gratitude (2 Kings 5). These stories illustrate that thankfulness is not just an emotional response—it's an act of faith that invites God's healing presence.

For the modern believer, these stories remind us that a grateful heart is a pathway to both spiritual renewal and physical vitality. But why? Gratitude aligns us with God's will, shifts our perspective from lack to abundance, and cultivates a peace that surpasses understanding—a peace that science now links to improved physical health.

The Science of Gratitude: A Modern Validation of Biblical Wisdom

Modern research provides a fascinating glimpse into how gratitude works on the body. Studies reveal that grateful individuals enjoy better physical health, lower levels of inflammation, and longer lifespans. Here's how science supports the transformative power of gratitude:

1. **Neurochemical Rewiring:** Gratitude stimulates the brain's reward centers, releasing serotonin and dopamine. These "feel-good" chemicals not only enhance mood but also reduce stress hormones like cortisol, which are harmful in excess.
2. **Immune System Strengthening:** A 2015 study found that people who practice gratitude regularly show increased natural killer cell activity, which is crucial for fighting infections and even cancer.
3. **Heart Health Benefits:** Research has demonstrated that gratitude lowers blood pressure and improves heart rate variability, reducing the risk of heart disease—the leading cause of death worldwide.
4. **Cellular Longevity:** Chronic stress accelerates cellular aging, but gratitude has the opposite effect. By promoting relaxation and emotional balance, gratitude protects telomeres—the caps on our DNA strands responsible for cellular repair and longevity.

These scientific findings don't just validate gratitude as a "nice-to-have" emotion. They show that it's a God-designed mechanism for physical and emotional resilience.

Faith: The Anchor for Emotional and Physical Health

Faith and gratitude go hand in hand, forming a virtuous cycle that reinforces well-being. Faith brings hope, and gratitude amplifies it, creating a sense of purpose that fuels resilience during life's hardest moments.

Faith isn't just about belief; it's about trust—trust in a plan greater than our own. When we surrender to God's sovereignty, our bodies respond with calm rather than chaos. Studies on people of faith show consistent links to:

- **Lower Anxiety and Depression Rates:** Faith fosters a sense of connection and purpose, reducing feelings of isolation that often lead to depression.
- **Improved Pain Tolerance:** Prayer and faith practices have been shown to alter perceptions of pain, making it more manageable.
- **Reduced Risk of Chronic Illness:** Believers tend to adopt healthier lifestyles and coping mechanisms, directly impacting physical health.

Biblical examples abound. Abraham trusted God's promise for a son despite his advanced age. His faith brought him joy, hope, and a legacy. Similarly, Jesus' healing miracles often included a phrase like, "Your faith has made you well" (Luke 17:19). Faith was not merely spiritual but an active agent in physical restoration.

Practical Steps to Cultivate Faith and Gratitude Daily

Building a lifestyle of faith and gratitude doesn't happen overnight—it's a daily practice. Start small and allow the habit to grow. Here are practical, scripture-rooted ways to begin:

- **Morning Gratitude Ritual:** Begin each day with a prayer of thanksgiving. Reflect on three things God has provided, no matter how small.
- **Scripture Journaling:** Write down Bible verses that emphasize thankfulness, such as Psalm 100:4 ("Enter his gates with thanksgiving and his courts with praise") and Philippians 4:6-7. Pair them with personal reflections.
- **Thanksgiving Walks:** Take time to walk outdoors, observing God's creation. Use this time to speak or silently reflect on blessings in your life.
- **Gratitude in Challenges:** When faced with hardship, follow Paul's example and give thanks. Write down what the challenge is teaching you or how it could deepen your faith.
- **Faith-Fueled Prayer Practices:** Dedicate a portion of your day to prayer that focuses on surrender and trust in God's plan.

These practices are not only spiritually enriching but also physically transformative. By creating a gratitude and faith routine, you activate God's design for a healthier, more joyful life.

Gratitude, Faith, and the Gift of Longevity

Faith and gratitude are divine tools for a longer, more meaningful life. They provide strength in adversity, joy in the mundane, and hope in the uncertain. Together, they form the foundation of biblical wellness. When you embrace gratitude and faith, you do more than survive—you thrive, living out the abundant life promised by Jesus: "I have come that they may have life, and have it to the full" (John 10:10).

In the end, a faith-filled, grateful life isn't just about adding years—it's about filling those years with purpose, joy, and peace.

GOD'S ANTI-AGING PLAN HIDDEN IN SCRIPTURE

Imagine unlocking a divine blueprint for vitality—one designed by God Himself and encoded in scripture. While modern society spends billions on anti-aging fads, the Bible quietly reveals timeless principles for living longer, stronger, and with greater joy. God's plan for vitality doesn't come in a pill but through rest, nourishment, faith, and movement—each working in perfect harmony to renew your body and spirit.

Rest, for example, is often dismissed in today's busy world, yet it's central to God's design for health. From the very beginning, God emphasized rest, blessing the seventh day and commanding us to follow His rhythm. Sleep and Sabbath aren't just spiritual acts; they're physical necessities. When you rest, your body engages in deep repair: your brain clears toxins, cells regenerate, and the immune system strengthens. Without rest, chronic stress accelerates aging and disease. By honoring God's command to rest, you not only honor Him but give your body the renewal it desperately needs.

Nourishment is another cornerstone of God's anti-aging plan. Genesis 1:29 provides the foundation: "I have given you every seed-bearing plant… They will be yours for food." These foods are more than sustenance—they are nature's original superfoods. Consider:

- **Figs:** Rich in antioxidants, figs fight free radicals that damage cells.
- **Pomegranates:** Known to improve heart health and enhance skin vitality.
- **Olive Oil:** A biblical staple with anti-inflammatory properties, promoting longevity.
- **Honey:** Called "good for the soul" in Proverbs, honey boosts energy and heals the body.

Incorporating these biblical foods into your diet doesn't just nourish your body—it aligns you with God's design for vitality and health.

But God's plan isn't limited to what you eat; it extends into your spiritual life. Faith and prayer are vital components of longevity. They don't just bring peace to your soul; they transform your body. Studies show that faith lowers cortisol levels (the stress hormone), improves heart health, and even slows cellular aging. Prayer acts as a release valve for burdens and a way to center your life on God's promises. Take Hezekiah, who prayed fervently and was granted 15 additional years of life. His story is a reminder that faith is a powerful force—not just spiritually but physically.

Movement also plays a crucial role in God's anti-aging plan. The Bible is full of examples of purposeful physical activity, from shepherds walking miles to tend flocks to builders laboring on God's temples. These acts weren't just work; they were acts of worship. Today, science confirms what scripture illustrates: regular physical activity strengthens muscles and bones, improves heart health, and keeps the mind sharp. The key is to embrace movement as part of a meaningful, God-centered life. Walk in nature as Jesus did, dance with joy like David, or engage in practical tasks like gardening, which connect you to creation.

To bring God's anti-aging plan into your daily life, consider these steps:

1. **Honor Rest:** Set aside a day each week to unplug, reflect, and reconnect with God. Prioritize quality sleep by creating a peaceful bedtime routine.
2. **Eat Intentionally:** Incorporate one biblical superfood into your meals each day—start with a drizzle of olive oil or a handful of figs.
3. **Pray with Purpose:** Begin and end each day with gratitude, thanking God for your body and asking for His guidance in caring for it.
4. **Move with Meaning:** Find ways to include joyful, intentional movement into your routine, like walking, stretching, or light physical labor.

God's anti-aging plan is simple, profound, and effective. It doesn't just add years to your life—it fills those years with vitality, joy, and purpose. By resting, nourishing, moving, and praying as scripture guides, you align yourself with the Creator's timeless wisdom, living not just longer but better.

LIVE LONGER WITH PURPOSE AND JOY EVERY DAY

What if the secret to a longer, fuller life wasn't locked away in a lab but hidden in plain sight—woven into scripture and waiting for us to embrace it? Living longer is about more than just adding years to your life; it's about filling those years with meaning, joy, and alignment with God's purpose. The Bible provides profound wisdom for cultivating this type of vibrant, purpose-driven living, and it begins with a mindset rooted in faith, gratitude, and intentionality.

The Power of Purpose: God's Design for a Meaningful Life

Purpose is a powerful force. It provides clarity in the face of chaos, motivation in moments of struggle, and a reason to keep going when life feels heavy. Scripture reinforces this truth time and again. Jeremiah 29:11 reminds us: "For I know the plans I have for you… plans to prosper you and not to harm you, plans to give you hope and a future." Living with purpose isn't just emotionally fulfilling—it's physically transformative.

Modern research confirms that people with a strong sense of purpose tend to live longer, healthier lives. Purpose lowers stress levels, reduces inflammation, and improves heart health. It gives the body a reason to thrive. In biblical terms, purpose is more than a goal—it's a calling. When we align our lives with God's design, we find strength and energy that surpasses human understanding.

Take Moses, for example. Called to lead God's people out of Egypt, Moses' life was far from easy, yet his purpose sustained him through trials. Despite immense challenges, Moses lived to the age of 120, his vigor intact to the end (Deuteronomy 34:7). This wasn't just biology; it was the strength of a life lived in alignment with God's will.

Joy: The Lifeblood of Longevity

Joy is more than fleeting happiness; it's a deep, abiding sense of peace and delight that comes from trusting God. The Bible often connects joy with strength: "The joy of the Lord is your strength" (Nehemiah 8:10). This isn't just metaphorical. Joy has profound physical benefits, from boosting the immune system to enhancing cardiovascular health and even improving cognitive function.

But how do we cultivate joy in a world filled with challenges? Scripture provides a roadmap:

- **Gratitude:** "Give thanks in all circumstances" (1 Thessalonians 5:18). Gratitude shifts your focus from what's missing to what's already abundant.
- **Trust in God:** "Cast all your anxiety on Him because He cares for you" (1 Peter 5:7). Surrendering your worries invites peace and joy to take their place.
- **Service to Others:** "It is more blessed to give than to receive" (Acts 20:35). Acts of kindness create joy that is both immediate and enduring.

The joy described in scripture isn't dependent on circumstances. It's a gift of the Spirit that sustains us through life's highs and lows. This joy not only enriches your days but also strengthens your body, enhancing resilience and longevity.

Practical Steps for Living with Purpose and Joy

Living a life filled with purpose and joy isn't something that happens by accident. It requires intentionality and a commitment to aligning your daily actions with God's wisdom. Here are steps to help you cultivate both:

1. **Define Your God-Given Purpose:** Spend time in prayer, asking God to reveal His calling for your life. Reflect on how your unique gifts and passions can serve His kingdom.
2. **Focus on Relationships:** Invest in meaningful connections with family, friends, and your faith community. Strong relationships are linked to longer, healthier lives.
3. **Celebrate Small Blessings:** Start each day by listing three things you're grateful for, no matter how small. Gratitude rewires your brain for joy.
4. **Prioritize Joyful Activities:** Incorporate practices that bring you genuine delight—whether it's singing, dancing, or spending time in nature. Make joy a daily habit.
5. **Trust in God's Timing:** Let go of striving and trust that God's plans are perfect. This trust will free you from unnecessary stress, allowing peace and joy to flourish.

When you live with purpose and joy, you create a life that radiates vitality. You wake up each day not just surviving but thriving, knowing that your time is being spent on what truly matters.

A Life Worth Living

Living longer with purpose and joy isn't just about improving your quality of life—it's about fulfilling the life God intended for you. Every breath you take is part of His divine plan, and when you embrace that truth, you unlock a life of profound meaning. By aligning your actions with His purpose and cultivating joy in every moment, you're not just adding years to your life—you're adding life to your years.

Are you ready to step into the vibrant, purpose-filled life God designed for you? The path is clear, and the tools are already in your hands. Let today be the day you begin living not just longer but better, with purpose and joy lighting your way.

BIBLICAL BRAIN HACKS FOR TOTAL PEACE

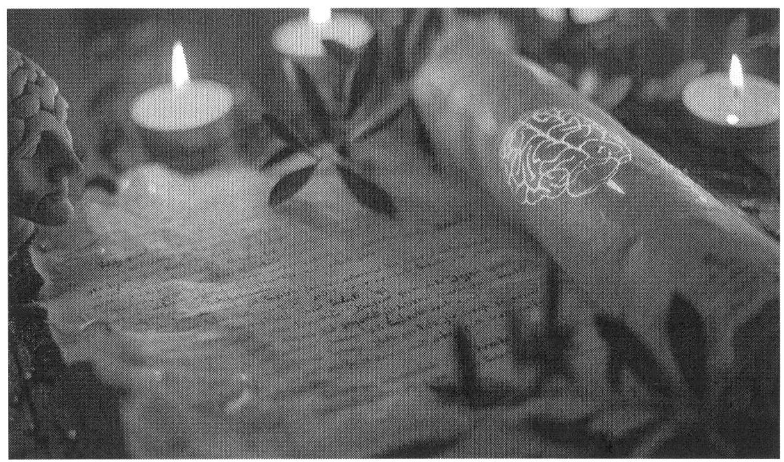

Imagine a life where your mind feels calm, focused, and free from the constant noise of worry and distraction. The Bible offers profound wisdom on achieving mental clarity and peace, providing tools that modern neuroscience is only beginning to validate. Scripture isn't just spiritual guidance—it's a blueprint for emotional resilience and mental well-being. Proverbs 3:5-6 tells us to "Trust in the Lord with all your heart and lean not on your own understanding." This verse speaks to a powerful truth: when we surrender our burdens to God, we release ourselves from the toxic grip of stress and anxiety, paving the way for mental clarity and lasting peace.

Practical applications of biblical brain hacks are surprisingly simple yet transformative. Daily prayer and meditation on scripture can quiet the racing mind and refocus your thoughts on God's promises. Repeating breath prayers like "Be still and know that I am God" (Psalm 46:10) aligns your breathing with a calm, meditative rhythm, reducing stress hormones and fostering emotional balance. Pair this with nourishing foods from scripture, such as walnuts and honey—brain-boosting superfoods mentioned in biblical texts—and you create a holistic approach to mental well-being. By trusting God and following these timeless practices, you can reclaim peace, strengthen focus, and find the rest your soul has been yearning for.

GOD'S BLUEPRINT FOR A CALM AND FOCUSED MIND

In today's chaotic world, a calm and focused mind often feels out of reach. The endless demands of work, relationships, and responsibilities can leave us feeling mentally drained and emotionally unbalanced. Yet, the Bible offers a powerful solution—a divine blueprint for achieving unshakable peace and clarity, no matter the circumstances. Isaiah 26:3 promises, "You will keep in perfect peace those whose minds are steadfast because they trust in you." This isn't just poetic comfort; it's a reminder that peace begins with trust in God and a mind fixed on His truth.

When your mind is anchored in faith, you're no longer swayed by fear, anxiety, or doubt. The Bible calls us to actively shift our focus from worry to worship, from panic to prayer. Take Philippians 4:6-7: "Do not be anxious about anything, but in every situation, by prayer and petition, with thanksgiving, present your requests to God. And the peace of God, which transcends all understanding, will guard your hearts and your minds in Christ Jesus." These verses reveal that peace isn't passive—it's cultivated through deliberate trust and communication with God.

Biblical Practices for Mental Clarity

God's blueprint for a calm mind is both spiritual and practical. Scripture outlines simple yet profound practices that can transform how you think and feel each day:

- **Meditate on God's Word:** Verses like Psalm 119:165 remind us, "Great peace have those who love your law." Reflecting on scripture quiets the racing mind and replaces worry with assurance.
- **Pray with Surrender:** Prayer isn't just asking for help—it's a moment to hand over your burdens to God. When you release control, you free your mind from the weight of overthinking.
- **Focus on Gratitude:** Gratitude shifts your mental perspective. By thanking God for what you have, you create a mindset of abundance rather than lack.
- **Breathe in His Presence:** Use breath prayers, like "Be still and know that I am God" (Psalm 46:10). These short prayers align your breathing with God's peace, calming your body and mind.

These practices not only ground you spiritually but also create mental habits that break the cycle of anxiety and distraction.

How to Bring God's Blueprint Into Your Life

Living with a calm and focused mind begins with small, intentional steps that connect you to God's wisdom. Start each morning by meditating on a verse that sets the tone for your day. Carry it with you, repeating it in moments of stress to recenter your thoughts. Build prayer breaks into your daily routine, even if it's just a quiet moment to speak with God. And before bed, reflect on your blessings and surrender any lingering worries into His hands.

By following these steps, you align your thoughts with God's eternal truths, creating a mind that is not only calm but resilient. You'll find yourself responding to life's challenges with clarity, focus, and peace—proof of God's promise that "perfect peace" comes to those who trust in Him.

<u>TRANSFORM YOUR MENTAL HEALTH WITH SCRIPTURE</u>

What if the most powerful mental health solutions weren't found in self-help books or therapy sessions but in the pages of the Bible? Scripture isn't just a source of spiritual guidance—it's a practical manual for emotional resilience and mental well-being. In a world that constantly pulls us into anxiety, stress, and fear, the Bible provides timeless strategies to restore peace and clarity. Philippians 4:6-7 offers this profound promise: "Do not be anxious about anything, but in every situation, by prayer and petition, with thanksgiving, present your requests to God. And the peace of God, which transcends all understanding, will guard your hearts and your minds in Christ Jesus." This verse gives us a step-by-step formula for mental health: pray, give thanks, and trust God to carry your burdens.

One of the most remarkable aspects of scripture is its ability to rewire how we think. Romans 12:2 commands us to "be transformed by the renewing of your mind." This isn't just metaphorical; it's an invitation to replace negative thought patterns with God's truth. When we meditate on His promises, our minds shift from chaos to calm, from fear to faith. Consider the Psalms, which were often written in times of distress yet continually return to themes of God's faithfulness and provision. Reflecting on verses like Psalm 34:17—"The righteous cry out, and the Lord hears them; He delivers them from all their troubles"—anchors your mind in hope and reminds you that no situation is beyond God's reach.

Practical Ways to Transform Your Thoughts with Scripture

The Bible equips us with tools to take control of our thoughts and emotions. These practices are simple but profoundly effective:

- **Replace Worry with Prayer:** Every time a worry enters your mind, use it as a trigger to pray. Turn your concerns into a conversation with God, knowing He hears every word.
- **Meditate on Key Verses:** Write down verses that resonate with you and revisit them throughout the day. Let their truth shape your thinking.

- **Use Affirmations from God's Word:** Replace negative self-talk with affirmations rooted in scripture, such as "I can do all things through Christ who strengthens me" (Philippians 4:13).
- **Speak Gratitude Out Loud:** Start and end your day by thanking God for specific blessings. Gratitude shifts your mindset from scarcity to abundance.
- **Practice Stillness in God's Presence:** Find a quiet space to sit and breathe deeply, focusing on verses like Psalm 46:10: "Be still and know that I am God."

By intentionally applying these practices, you can retrain your mind to focus on God's promises instead of your problems. Over time, this daily discipline transforms how you respond to challenges, building resilience and peace.

The Ripple Effect of a Transformed Mind

When you apply these scriptural principles, the transformation doesn't just stay in your mind—it overflows into every area of your life. You'll notice better relationships, more clarity in decision-making, and a greater ability to handle stress. Even science confirms the benefits: prayer and meditation reduce cortisol (the stress hormone), improve heart health, and create lasting emotional stability.

But beyond these benefits lies something even more profound: a deeper connection with God. When your thoughts align with His truth, you no longer feel weighed down by the world's demands. Instead, you walk in freedom, knowing that His peace guards your heart and mind. Transforming your mental health with scripture isn't just about survival—it's about thriving in the life God has called you to live.

Are you ready to embrace the peace and clarity God promises? Start today by committing your thoughts to Him, one verse at a time. The transformation begins the moment you surrender your mind to His Word.

FOODS THAT SHARPEN THE MIND AND UPLIFT THE SPIRIT

The Bible reveals not only spiritual truths but also practical wisdom for nourishing the body and mind. Among its pages are references to foods that are not only good for your health but also for your mental clarity and emotional well-being. Modern science is just beginning to uncover what scripture has known all along: the foods God designed are powerful tools for a sharp mind and a joyful spirit. Proverbs 24:13 advises, "Eat honey, my son, for it is good; honey from the comb is sweet to your taste." This simple verse highlights how natural foods can refresh and energize both body and soul.

Many of the foods mentioned in scripture are rich in nutrients essential for brain health. Walnuts, for example, are often associated with wisdom in ancient texts and resemble the shape of the brain—a fitting coincidence for a food packed with omega-3 fatty acids, which improve cognitive function. Honey, described as a symbol of abundance and sweetness, provides quick energy and antioxidants to fight inflammation in the brain. Other biblical staples, such as figs and pomegranates, are loaded with vitamins and antioxidants that promote mental clarity and protect against the cognitive decline associated with aging. Olive oil, frequently referred to as "liquid gold" in biblical times, nourishes the brain with healthy fats that support memory and focus.

How to Incorporate Biblical Superfoods into Your Diet

God's design for food is simple, pure, and life-giving. To sharpen your mind and uplift your spirit, start by bringing these scripture-endorsed foods into your daily meals:

- **Walnuts:** Add a handful to your morning oatmeal or salad for a brain-boosting dose of healthy fats and antioxidants.
- **Honey:** Use it to sweeten herbal tea or drizzle over whole-grain toast for sustained energy without the crash of processed sugars.
- **Olive Oil:** Replace processed oils with extra virgin olive oil when cooking or as a dressing for salads to support cognitive function.
- **Figs:** Enjoy them as a snack or pair them with cheese for a naturally sweet, nutrient-packed treat.
- **Pomegranates:** Use the seeds as a topping for yogurt, salads, or even roasted vegetables for a burst of flavor and brain-protecting antioxidants.

Each of these foods is a gift from God, designed to fuel not just your body but your mind. By eating as God intended, you align your physical and mental health with His perfect design.

The Spiritual and Emotional Power of Nourishment

Eating isn't just a physical act—it's deeply spiritual. When you choose foods that honor God's creation, you're engaging in a sacred act of stewardship over your body. The Bible reminds us that our bodies are temples of the Holy Spirit (1 Corinthians 6:19), and what we put into them affects not only our health but also our ability to serve God with energy and clarity.

Moreover, the act of preparing and consuming these foods can be an opportunity for gratitude and reflection. As you nourish your body with these brain-sharpening, spirit-lifting foods, take time to thank God for His provision and wisdom. With each bite, you're not just feeding yourself; you're equipping your mind and soul to live out His purpose with focus and joy.

Are you ready to embrace God's wisdom for a sharper, more joyful mind? Start today by incorporating these sacred foods into your life and experience the transformation they bring.

SIMPLE PRAYERS AND PRACTICES TO ERASE ANXIETY

Anxiety has a way of gripping even the strongest hearts, clouding your mind and stealing your peace. But the Bible offers an antidote: simple yet powerful prayers and practices that allow you to hand your burdens to God and invite His peace into your life. Psalm 55:22 declares, "Cast your cares on the Lord, and He will sustain you; He will never let the righteous be shaken." This isn't just spiritual encouragement—it's a call to action. The key to erasing anxiety lies in surrendering your fears to God and trusting Him to carry them.

Prayer is one of the most effective ways to calm an anxious heart. Breath prayers, in particular, are simple and grounding, helping you refocus on God's promises while quieting the chaos within. These short, repetitive prayers align with your breathing, creating a sense of stillness and trust. Here are a few to try:

- **"Be still and know that I am God"** (Psalm 46:10) – A reminder of God's control in every situation.
- **"Cast all your anxiety on Him because He cares for you"** (1 Peter 5:7) – A release of burdens into God's loving hands.
- **"The Lord is my shepherd; I lack nothing"** (Psalm 23:1) – A declaration of trust in God's provision.
- **"Peace I leave with you; my peace I give you"** (John 14:27) – A powerful affirmation of the peace Christ offers.
- **"The Lord is my light and my salvation—whom shall I fear?"** (Psalm 27:1) – A declaration of confidence in God's protection.
- **"Do not fear, for I am with you; do not be dismayed, for I am your God."** (Isaiah 41:10) – A reminder of God's constant presence and strength.
- **"Create in me a clean heart, O God, and renew a steadfast spirit within me."** (Psalm 51:10) – A plea for renewal and peace.
- **"I can do all things through Christ who strengthens me."** (Philippians 4:13) – An affirmation of resilience through Christ's power.
- **"When I am afraid, I put my trust in You."** (Psalm 56:3) – A simple act of surrender in moments of fear.
- **"Come to me, all you who are weary and burdened, and I will give you rest."** (Matthew 11:28) – An invitation to find rest in Jesus.

Pair these prayers with the practice of gratitude, as instructed in Philippians 4:6-7: "Do not be anxious about anything, but in every situation, by prayer and petition, with thanksgiving, present your requests to God." Gratitude reshapes your perspective, shifting your focus from fear to faith. Each day, write down three things you're thankful for, and reflect on how God's hand has been present in your life.

Practical Ways to Incorporate Peaceful Practices

These prayers and practices are most effective when integrated into your daily life. Start small, building moments of prayer and stillness into your routine:

- **Morning Prayer:** Begin each day with a centering prayer, asking God for peace and clarity as you face the day ahead.
- **Midday Gratitude Check:** Pause halfway through the day to list three blessings you've noticed, thanking God for His provision.
- **Evening Reflection:** Before bed, release your worries to God in prayer and meditate on His promises of peace.

Anxiety doesn't have the final word when you anchor your heart in God's truth. Through prayer, gratitude, and trust, you can invite His peace to guard your mind and transform your days into moments of calm, joy, and assurance.

GOD'S RHYTHM HACK TO BEAT MODERN CHAOS

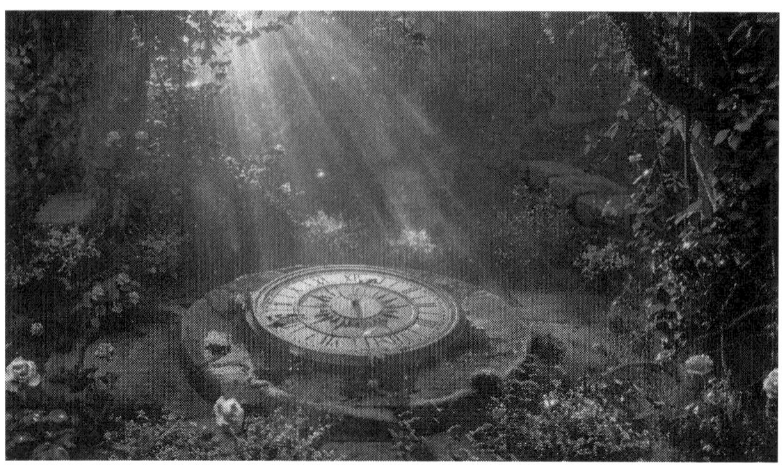

In the relentless pace of modern life, where deadlines, distractions, and demands never seem to end, it's easy to feel disconnected, overwhelmed, and out of sync. Yet, God's Word reveals an ancient, divine rhythm for living—a pattern of work, rest, and worship designed to restore balance and harmony to our lives. This rhythm isn't just a spiritual ideal; it's a practical framework for thriving in the midst of chaos. From the cycles of creation to the gift of the Sabbath, scripture reminds us that when we align with God's natural rhythms, we don't just survive the noise of life—we rise above it with peace, clarity, and purpose. This chapter explores how you can reclaim that rhythm and experience the transformative power of living according to God's design.

<u>HOW TO ALIGN YOUR LIFE WITH DIVINE RHYTHMS</u>

Life today often feels like a relentless race, where the finish line keeps moving and the demands never seem to end. But what if there was a way to step off the treadmill of modern chaos and find lasting peace? The Bible provides a clear answer: aligning your life with God's divine rhythms. From the very beginning, God set a pattern for humanity to follow, modeling balance through His creation. Genesis 2:2-3 tells us, "By the seventh day, God had finished the work He had been doing; so on the seventh day He rested… Then God blessed the seventh day and made it holy." This rhythm of work, rest, and worship wasn't just for Him—it was a gift and a guide for us.

God's rhythms are designed to restore us physically, mentally, and spiritually. When we follow His patterns, we step into a life of purpose and peace rather than exhaustion and anxiety. The Sabbath, for instance, isn't merely a day off; it's a sacred pause to reconnect with God and realign our priorities. It's a time to let go of striving and remember that our value doesn't come from what we produce but from who we are in Him. By honoring this rhythm, we regain clarity and strength for the work ahead, just as the Israelites did when God instructed them to rest after their six days of gathering manna in the wilderness (Exodus 16:26-30).

Practical Steps to Align with God's Rhythms

To live in harmony with divine rhythms, you don't need to overhaul your life overnight. Start with small, intentional changes that create space for rest, reflection, and connection with God:

- **Set Aside a Sabbath:** Choose one day a week to unplug from work, chores, and distractions. Use this time to pray, reflect, and enjoy restorative activities that draw you closer to God.
- **Embrace Morning Devotionals:** Begin each day with a few moments of scripture and prayer. This morning rhythm sets a tone of peace and purpose for the day ahead.
- **Establish a Work-Rest Balance:** Follow God's pattern by setting clear boundaries between work and rest. Avoid overloading your schedule and prioritize downtime to recharge.
- **Live Seasonally:** Recognize the rhythms of nature as part of God's design. Reflect on how the seasons mirror cycles of growth, harvest, rest, and renewal in your own life.
- **Incorporate Daily Worship:** Whether through prayer, singing, or quiet reflection, weave moments of worship into your day to stay connected to God's presence.

Each of these steps aligns your actions with the natural flow of life as God intended, fostering a deeper sense of balance and fulfillment.

The Peace and Power of Divine Rhythms

When you live according to God's rhythms, you'll notice a profound shift in how you approach life's challenges. You'll experience less burnout and more clarity, fewer distractions and deeper focus. The world's pace may feel relentless, but God invites you into a life that is steady, intentional, and deeply satisfying. As Jesus said in Matthew 11:28-29, "Come to me, all you who are weary and burdened, and I will give you rest… For my yoke is easy, and my burden is light." Aligning with divine rhythms is about stepping into that rest—where you work diligently, rest fully, and live joyfully, all within the framework of God's perfect design.

SEASONAL LIVING: HONORING GOD'S NATURAL CYCLES

What if the secret to a more balanced, joyful life was hidden in the rhythm of the seasons themselves? God's creation is a masterpiece of cycles—spring's renewal, summer's abundance, autumn's harvest, and winter's rest. These aren't just random occurrences; they're divine whispers calling us to align with His timing. Ecclesiastes 3:1 proclaims, "There is a time for everything, and a season for every activity under the heavens." Yet, in today's 24/7 world, we've lost touch with this sacred rhythm, living as if every season demands the same energy, pace, and output.

The Israelites understood the power of seasonal living. Their lives were intimately connected to God's natural cycles. Planting and harvesting were spiritual acts, intertwined with celebrations like Passover and the Feast of Tabernacles, which praised God's provision. These rhythms were more than agricultural—they were deeply restorative, reminding God's people when to work, when to celebrate, and when to rest. Contrast this with our modern reality: endless deadlines, artificial lighting, and an unrelenting pace that defies God's natural order. Could it be that our disconnection from the seasons is at the root of our exhaustion and anxiety?

How to Reconnect with God's Rhythms

The good news is that God's cycles are still waiting to guide us back to balance. By living seasonally, you can rediscover the peace and purpose that come from moving in harmony with His creation. Here's how:

- **Spring: A Time for Renewal** – As the earth awakens, so should your spirit. Use this season to plant seeds of growth—new habits, deeper faith, or long-overdue goals. Reflect on Isaiah 43:19: "See, I am doing a new thing! Now it springs up; do you not perceive it?"
- **Summer: A Time for Abundance** – Celebrate the fullness of life. Spend time outdoors, enjoy the fruits of your labor, and soak in God's blessings. Like the Psalmist, declare, "The earth is full of the goodness of the Lord" (Psalm 33:5).
- **Autumn: A Time for Gratitude** – As the harvest comes in, take stock of the blessings in your life. This is the season to prepare for the months ahead, storing up not just provisions but a heart full of thankfulness. "Give thanks to the Lord, for He is good; His love endures forever" (1 Chronicles 16:34).
- **Winter: A Time for Rest** – Embrace stillness. This is a sacred season for reflection and restoration, a time to trust that God is working even when life feels dormant. Remember Psalm 37:7: "Be still before the Lord and wait patiently for Him."

The Sacred Gift of Seasonal Living

Living seasonally isn't just about planting gardens or observing weather changes—it's about letting the seasons of your life reflect God's divine order. We all experience springs of growth, summers of joy, autumns of transition, and winters of waiting. Each season carries its own beauty and lessons, reminding us that God's timing is perfect.

When you honor these cycles, something remarkable happens: the frantic pace of modern life fades, replaced by a sense of flow and purpose. You learn to embrace rest without guilt, to celebrate without hesitation, and to trust God's plan, even in the quieter seasons. You'll find that life isn't just something to endure—it's a divine rhythm to dance to.

Are you ready to tune your life to God's seasons? Start by slowing down, paying attention to His creation, and letting each season guide your heart back to Him.

CREATE DAILY ROUTINES THAT REFLECT GOD'S WISDOM

What if the secret to a peaceful, fulfilling life wasn't in doing more but in structuring your days around God's divine wisdom? The Bible offers a framework for daily living that promotes balance, clarity, and purpose. By designing routines that honor God's rhythms of work, rest, and worship, you can transform even the most ordinary day into a sacred journey. Psalm 90:12 urges us, "Teach us to number our days, that we may gain a heart of wisdom." This verse reminds us that time is a gift, and how we spend it matters deeply.

God's wisdom is clear: our days aren't meant to be endless cycles of busyness and exhaustion. From morning to night, we are invited to live intentionally, weaving in moments of prayer, gratitude, and rest. Consider the example of Jesus, whose ministry was filled with purpose yet never chaotic. He often withdrew to solitary places to pray (Luke 5:16), showing us the importance of quiet reflection in the midst of a full life. By modeling your daily routines after this divine example, you can create a life that is not only productive but also deeply fulfilling.

Steps to Build a God-Centered Daily Routine

Designing a routine that honors God doesn't require radical changes—it starts with small, deliberate steps. Here are ways to align your day with His wisdom:

- **Morning:** Begin your day with gratitude and focus. Spend the first few moments in prayer or meditation on scripture. Verses like Psalm

118:24—"This is the day that the Lord has made; let us rejoice and be glad in it"—set a positive and intentional tone.

- **Midday:** Take a break to reconnect with God. A simple prayer or moment of reflection during lunch can reset your mindset and remind you of His presence in your work.
- **Evening:** End your day by surrendering your worries and thanking God for His faithfulness. Reflect on 1 Peter 5:7: "Cast all your anxiety on Him because He cares for you."

Infuse Purpose Into the Everyday

Your routine doesn't need to feel rigid or overwhelming—it should flow naturally, creating space for God to guide your actions. Incorporate faith into ordinary tasks. For example, use cooking as a time for gratitude, thanking God for the nourishment He provides. Turn household chores into acts of worship by playing hymns or reflecting on scripture while you work. These small shifts turn the mundane into meaningful, connecting your everyday life to God's greater purpose.

The Beauty of Living in God's Rhythm

When you create routines that reflect God's wisdom, you'll notice a profound shift. Stress begins to fade, replaced by a sense of balance and clarity. You'll wake up with a renewed focus and go to bed with a heart full of gratitude. Life no longer feels like a race but a deliberate walk with God, where every step is guided by His hand. By aligning your daily routines with His design, you honor Him, find peace, and live with purpose.

Are you ready to reshape your days and discover the beauty of living in sync with God's wisdom? Start small, trust the process, and watch as your life transforms into one that reflects His peace and glory.

THE SACRED HEALING PLAN NO ONE TAUGHT YOU

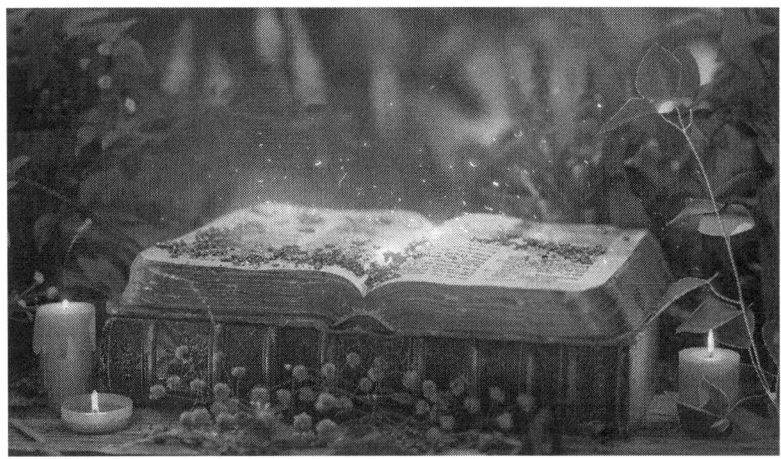

Hidden within the pages of the Bible lies a powerful, life-changing blueprint for healing—a plan that modern medicine has largely overlooked. This sacred healing plan is not about quick fixes or temporary relief but about achieving true wellness by aligning your physical, emotional, and spiritual health with God's design. Throughout scripture, we see God's wisdom guiding His people to practices that restore vitality and foster peace, from the power of prayer and gratitude to the healing properties of natural remedies and rest. This chapter will unveil the holistic principles God embedded in His Word, showing you how to reclaim your health and thrive in ways you may have never thought possible. It's time to rediscover what God intended: a life of balance, healing, and divine alignment.

HOW SPIRITUAL HEALTH ANCHORS PHYSICAL WELLNESS

What if the key to vibrant physical health was rooted not just in diet and exercise but in the state of your soul? The Bible repeatedly emphasizes that our spiritual well-being is deeply intertwined with our physical vitality. Proverbs 4:20-22 declares, "My son, pay attention to what I say; turn your ear to my words. Do not let them out of your sight, keep them within your heart; for they are life to those who find them and health to one's whole body." This profound truth reveals that God's Word is more than spiritual guidance—it's a source of healing for the entire body.

When your spiritual health is strong, your physical body follows suit. Faith, prayer, and trust in God reduce stress, one of the greatest contributors to illness. Studies have shown that stress weakens the immune system, increases inflammation, and accelerates aging. But scripture provides an antidote. Verses like 1 Peter 5:7—"Cast all your anxiety on Him because He cares for you"—remind us to release our burdens to God. This act of surrender doesn't just ease the mind; it calms the body, lowering stress hormones like cortisol and promoting physical renewal.

The Science Behind Spiritual Wellness

Modern science is catching up with what scripture has long taught. Here's how spiritual practices improve physical health:

- **Prayer:** Regular prayer and meditation lower blood pressure, reduce inflammation, and boost immune function, creating a calmer, healthier body.
- **Gratitude:** Practicing gratitude, as the Bible instructs, activates the brain's reward system, releasing "feel-good" chemicals like serotonin and dopamine. These chemicals improve mood and help regulate bodily functions like digestion and sleep.
- **Community Worship:** Engaging in faith-based communities fosters connection and reduces feelings of loneliness, which has been linked to chronic illness and shortened lifespan.

These findings affirm what the Bible has always taught: a strong connection with God doesn't just heal the soul—it rejuvenates the body.

How to Strengthen Your Spiritual Core for Better Health

Aligning your spiritual health with physical wellness doesn't require monumental changes; it begins with simple, intentional steps. Here's how you can start:

- **Daily Prayer:** Begin and end each day by speaking with God. Share your worries, express gratitude, and ask for strength and healing.
- **Meditate on Scripture:** Reflect on verses that connect spiritual peace with physical health, such as Psalm 103:2-3: "Praise the Lord, my soul… who forgives all your sins and heals all your diseases."
- **Trust God's Timing:** Release control over situations that cause stress and anxiety. Trust that God's plan is perfect, even when it's hard to see.
- **Serve Others:** Acts of service shift your focus from your own struggles to the needs of others, fostering emotional and spiritual renewal that ripples through your body.

The Harmony of Body and Soul

When your spiritual health thrives, it anchors your physical wellness, creating harmony that transforms your entire being. You'll feel lighter, more energized, and better equipped to handle life's challenges. This is God's design: a life where the body, mind, and spirit work together in unity, reflecting His love and wisdom. By nurturing your soul, you unlock the physical vitality God intended for you—a vibrant life filled with purpose, peace, and strength.

BUILD HABITS ROOTED IN PRAYER AND GRATITUDE

Habits are the invisible architecture of our lives. They determine how we spend our days, respond to challenges, and ultimately grow closer to—or further from—God. The Bible repeatedly emphasizes the importance of intentional, God-centered habits, especially those rooted in prayer and gratitude. Colossians 4:2 advises, "Devote yourselves to prayer, being watchful and thankful." This isn't just spiritual advice—it's a call to cultivate practices that nourish your soul, anchor your mind, and even impact your physical health. When prayer and gratitude become daily habits, they transform the way you approach life, fostering resilience, peace, and joy that radiate into every corner of your being.

Prayer is more than a spiritual exercise; it's a lifeline that keeps you connected to God. Regular prayer cultivates humility, surrender, and trust, reminding us that we're not in control—and that's okay. It invites God into our lives, allowing His wisdom and strength to guide us. Meanwhile, gratitude shifts our perspective from scarcity to abundance, helping us recognize God's goodness even in the midst of challenges. Modern science supports the profound impact of these practices. Studies show that gratitude rewires the brain to focus on positive experiences, reducing anxiety and depression. Prayer, likewise, has been linked to lower blood pressure, improved mental clarity, and greater emotional stability. Together, prayer and gratitude form a powerful duo that aligns your mind, body, and spirit with God's design.

The Power of Consistent Prayer

Prayer is a habit that takes time to develop but yields extraordinary results. By dedicating specific moments of your day to prayer, you create a rhythm that keeps your heart aligned with God. Prayer is not about eloquence or perfection; it's about consistency and authenticity. The Bible gives us countless examples of prayer as a transformative practice, from Daniel praying three times a day (Daniel 6:10) to Jesus retreating to quiet places to pray (Luke 5:16). These examples teach us that prayer isn't just reactive; it's proactive—a habit that shapes your mindset before life's challenges arise.

To make prayer a daily habit, consider starting with these approaches:

- **Set a Time and Place:** Designate a consistent time and quiet space for prayer each day. Mornings work well for many, as they set the tone for the rest of the day.
- **Keep It Simple:** Start with short prayers, focusing on gratitude, requests for guidance, and moments of praise. Use the Lord's Prayer (Matthew 6:9-13) as a model if you're unsure where to begin.
- **Use Visual Prompts:** Place a sticky note with a prayer reminder on your bathroom mirror or kitchen counter to prompt you to pause and pray.

As you commit to prayer, you'll notice it becomes not just a practice but a source of strength and clarity. Over time, prayer will feel as natural and essential as breathing.

Gratitude: The Habit That Rewires Your Mind

Gratitude is more than saying "thank you"—it's an intentional mindset that transforms how you see the world. The Bible frequently links gratitude with peace and joy, as in 1 Thessalonians 5:16-18: "Rejoice always, pray continually, give thanks in all circumstances; for this is God's will for you in Christ Jesus." Gratitude helps you recognize God's presence and provision in your life, even in difficult seasons.

To make gratitude a daily habit, try these practical steps:

- **Start a Gratitude Journal:** Each morning, write down three things you're thankful for. Be specific—don't just say "family," but write "The time my daughter made me laugh yesterday." Specificity makes gratitude more powerful.
- **Turn Complaints into Thankfulness:** When you catch yourself complaining, pause and find something positive in the situation. For instance, instead of griping about a tough workday, thank God for the opportunity to grow through challenges.
- **Incorporate Gratitude into Meals:** Before eating, take a moment to thank God not just for the food but for His ongoing provision in your life.

Gratitude isn't always easy, especially in seasons of hardship. But it's in these moments that it becomes most transformative, shifting your focus from what you lack to what God has already provided.

Practical Habits to Combine Prayer and Gratitude

The true power of prayer and gratitude lies in how they work together. Prayer deepens your connection to God, while gratitude reshapes your perspective. Here are ways to integrate these practices into your daily life:

- **Morning Routine:** Start your day with a short prayer of thanks and a verse of scripture. Reflect on a specific blessing from the previous day and ask God for guidance in the day ahead.
- **Prayer Walks:** Take a short walk during your lunch break or in the evening, using the time to thank God for His creation and talk to Him about your worries or joys.
- **Gratitude Reminders:** Set an alarm on your phone during the day with a note that says, "Pause and thank God for three blessings right now."
- **Evening Reflection:** Before bed, spend five minutes in prayer, thanking God for specific moments from the day. End with a request for peace as you sleep and strength for tomorrow.

These simple habits weave prayer and gratitude into the fabric of your day, creating a rhythm that keeps you centered and connected to God.

The Transformative Impact of These Habits

When you build your life around prayer and gratitude, the transformation is undeniable. You'll find yourself less reactive and more reflective, better equipped to handle stress, and more attuned to the blessings around you. Gratitude shifts your focus from scarcity to abundance, while prayer reminds you of God's sovereignty and love. Together, these habits don't just improve your emotional and spiritual health—they ripple into your physical well-being, fostering resilience, joy, and a profound sense of peace.

This isn't about perfection—it's about progress. Each moment spent in prayer or gratitude brings you closer to a life rooted in God's wisdom and love, creating a foundation that no storm can shake.

CREATE A SACRED WELLNESS ROUTINE THAT HEALS

A truly transformative daily routine doesn't just cater to your physical needs—it nourishes your body, mind, and spirit in harmony with God's design. A sacred wellness routine is more than a checklist of tasks; it's a deliberate alignment of your daily actions with faith-centered principles that restore balance, foster gratitude, and deepen your connection to God. Rooted in scripture, this blueprint offers a step-by-step guide to creating a routine that renews you from the inside out, drawing on God's wisdom for holistic healing.

Morning: Begin with Purpose and Connection

How you start your day sets the tone for everything that follows. The Bible emphasizes the importance of seeking God early: "In the morning, Lord, you hear my voice; in the morning I lay my requests before you and wait expectantly"

(Psalm 5:3). Your morning routine should center on grounding yourself in faith and inviting God to guide your day.

1. **Gratitude Practice:** As soon as you wake, thank God for three specific blessings. This shifts your focus to His provision and sets a tone of abundance.
2. **Prayer and Reflection:** Spend 5-10 minutes in prayer, surrendering your plans to God and seeking His guidance. Use a scripture like Proverbs 3:5-6—"Trust in the Lord with all your heart and lean not on your own understanding."
3. **Scripture Meditation:** Read a passage of scripture and meditate on its application to your life. Use verses that bring encouragement or focus, such as Psalm 23 or Matthew 6:25-34.
4. **Movement:** Engage in gentle physical activity, such as stretching, yoga, or a brisk walk. As you move, reflect on the gift of your body and offer prayers of gratitude for your health.

Midday: Refresh and Reconnect

The middle of the day often brings stress and distractions, making it a crucial time to pause, recenter, and refuel. Jesus Himself withdrew from crowds to pray during busy days (Luke 5:16), demonstrating the importance of stepping away from life's demands to reconnect with God.

1. **Mindful Meal:** Use lunchtime as an opportunity to honor God's provision. Say a prayer of gratitude before eating and focus on enjoying nourishing, wholesome foods that reflect God's creation.
2. **Prayer Break:** Take five minutes to step away from work or daily tasks to pray. Use this time to release stress, ask for strength, and reflect on God's presence in your day.
3. **Reflection or Journaling:** Write down one or two things that have gone well so far and thank God for them. If challenges have arisen, surrender them to Him, trusting in His wisdom and timing.

Evening: Rest and Restore in God's Presence

The end of your day is a sacred opportunity to reflect, release, and rest in God's peace. Psalm 4:8 reminds us, "In peace I will lie down and sleep, for you alone, Lord, make me dwell in safety." Your evening routine should focus on letting go of the day's burdens and preparing your mind and body for restful sleep.

1. **Gratitude Review:** Reflect on the day and write down three moments or blessings you are grateful for. This practice helps you end the day with a positive and peaceful mindset.

2. **Evening Prayer:** Spend time in prayer, thanking God for His faithfulness throughout the day. Ask for forgiveness where needed and peace as you rest.
3. **Scripture or Devotional Reading:** Close your day by reading a passage of scripture or a devotional that reminds you of God's promises. Focus on verses about rest and renewal, such as Matthew 11:28-30.
4. **Wind-Down Routine:** Incorporate calming practices like deep breathing, quiet music, or journaling your thoughts. Let these activities center your heart on God as you prepare for sleep.

Weekly: Incorporate a Sabbath Rhythm

In addition to daily practices, God designed the Sabbath as a weekly opportunity for restoration and worship. Exodus 20:8 commands us to "Remember the Sabbath day by keeping it holy." Dedicate one day each week to unplugging from work, spending time with loved ones, and focusing on God. Use this time for extended prayer, scripture study, and activities that bring joy and renewal, such as spending time in nature or sharing a meal with family.

Customizing Your Sacred Wellness Routine

While this blueprint provides a foundation, your routine should reflect your unique needs and circumstances. Begin with small, manageable changes, and allow your routine to grow organically as you discover what nourishes your body, mind, and spirit. Whether it's adding a longer morning prayer time, incorporating scripture memorization, or adjusting your schedule for more physical movement, the goal is to align your actions with God's rhythms and intentions.

Over time, these practices will become second nature, transforming your routine into a sacred space where healing and growth flourish. With each prayer, each moment of gratitude, and each act of reflection, you'll find yourself living in greater harmony with God's plan—mind, body, and spirit united in His care.

BECOME THE KEEPER OF HIDDEN HEALING SECRETS

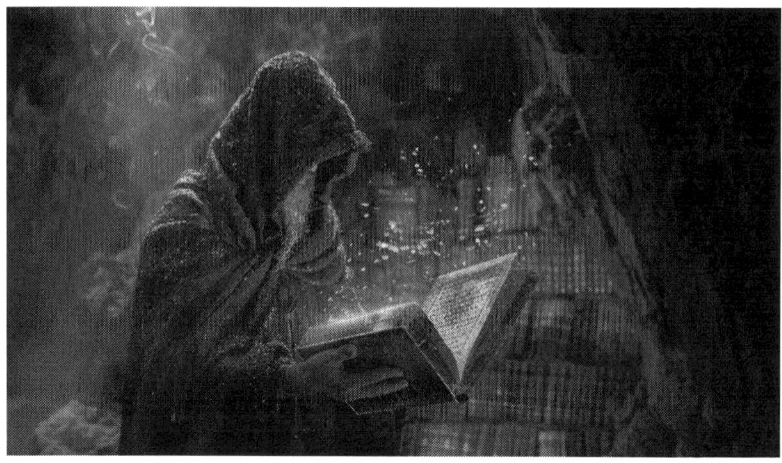

The journey through the hidden healing secrets of the Bible isn't just about transforming your own life—it's about carrying these timeless truths forward. As a keeper of this wisdom, you have the opportunity to embody God's design for health, wellness, and spiritual alignment, inspiring others to do the same. Proverbs 4:7 declares, "Wisdom is supreme; therefore get wisdom. Though it cost all you have, get understanding." By living out these principles, you become a light in a world that desperately needs healing, sharing the gift of biblical wellness with your family, community, and future generations. This closing chapter will empower you to take what you've learned and become a steward of God's ultimate healing blueprint, passing down these life-changing truths to those you love and ensuring they are never forgotten.

INSPIRE YOUR FAMILY TO LIVE FAITH-BASED WELLNESS

Imagine your home becoming a sanctuary of health, joy, and faith—a place where your family thrives not only physically but also spiritually. As the Bible teaches, true wellness begins with the heart and radiates outward, transforming relationships, routines, and even how we face challenges. Proverbs 22:6 reminds us, "Train up a child in the way he should go, and when he is old, he will not depart from it." When you lead your family in faith-based wellness, you're planting seeds that will bear fruit for generations to come.

The key to inspiring your family is leading by example. When they see you practicing gratitude, praying intentionally, and prioritizing rest and nourishment, they're more likely to follow suit. Make faith-centered wellness a family effort, weaving biblical principles into everyday activities. Mealtimes, for instance, can become sacred moments of connection and gratitude. Before eating, take a moment to pray together, thanking God not just for the food but for the hands that prepared it and the blessings of the day. Simple traditions like this create a ripple effect of mindfulness and joy.

Practical Ways to Bring Faith-Based Wellness Into Your Family's Life

- **Daily Family Prayer:** Set aside time to pray together as a family, whether it's in the morning, at dinner, or before bedtime. Rotate who leads the prayer to encourage participation and personal growth.
- **Shared Devotionals:** Choose a short Bible passage or devotional to read and discuss together. Reflect on how its message applies to your family's daily life.
- **Faith-Filled Activities:** Engage in activities that connect your family to God's creation, like gardening, hiking, or stargazing. Use these moments to marvel at His handiwork and discuss His presence in your lives.
- **Gratitude Challenges:** Make gratitude a fun and engaging family habit. Each person can share one thing they're thankful for at dinner or before bed. Even younger children can participate, fostering a positive mindset early on.
- **Sabbath Rest as a Family:** Dedicate one day a week to unplugging from work, screens, and distractions. Spend time worshiping, relaxing, and enjoying each other's company.

Create a Legacy of Faith and Health

Inspiring your family to live faith-based wellness isn't just about the here and now—it's about creating a legacy. As you model these principles, you're teaching your children, grandchildren, and loved ones that God's design for health is holistic, encompassing body, mind, and spirit. You're showing them that true wellness comes not from fleeting trends but from a foundation of trust in God's wisdom. Over time, these practices become ingrained, shaping how your family approaches life, health, and faith for generations.

Your role as a guide is more powerful than you may realize. Through your actions, your family will come to see wellness not as a chore but as an act of worship, a way to honor God and live abundantly. Let faith-based wellness become the heartbeat of your home—a source of healing, connection, and enduring love.

LIVE AS A SHINING EXAMPLE OF GOD'S HEALING PLAN

True transformation begins with you. When you embrace God's healing plan, your life becomes a living testimony of His wisdom, grace, and provision. As Matthew 5:16 urges, "Let your light shine before others, that they may see your good deeds and glorify your Father in heaven." By living as a shining example of faith-based wellness, you inspire others—not through words alone but through the undeniable power of your actions and the peace and vitality they bring.

Your daily choices speak volumes. When you prioritize rest, pray through life's challenges, and nourish your body as God intended, you radiate a sense of balance and joy that draws others in. People will begin to notice the way you approach life differently—the calm you bring to chaos, the gratitude you express in tough times, and the energy with which you engage in God's work. These outward expressions of wellness reflect the inward transformation of aligning your life with God's design.

Ways to Reflect God's Healing in Your Life

- **Radiate Peace:** Approach challenges with calm and trust, modeling what it means to cast your burdens on God (1 Peter 5:7). Your steadiness will inspire those around you to seek the same peace.
- **Prioritize Relationships:** Dedicate time to connecting with loved ones, showing them that faith-based wellness values community and love above busyness.
- **Lead with Gratitude:** Make gratitude a visible part of your life, thanking God openly for blessings big and small. This fosters a culture of thankfulness in your circle.
- **Invite Others to Join:** Share your faith-centered practices, whether it's a family prayer routine, a Sabbath tradition, or a favorite scripture. Openly explain how these habits have transformed your health and spirit.
- **Celebrate God's Creation:** Actively engage with the world God created—whether through gardening, enjoying nature walks, or cooking wholesome meals—and invite others to experience this joy with you.

Living as an example doesn't require perfection; it requires consistency and authenticity. People are drawn to the evidence of faith in action, not to unattainable ideals. When others see your life flourishing under God's guidance, they'll be inspired to explore His healing plan for themselves.

In a world that so often seeks quick fixes and temporary satisfaction, you have the opportunity to show a better way—a life rooted in God's eternal truths. By living faithfully, you not only reflect His healing plan but also invite others to join in its blessings. Together, your actions and faith create a ripple effect that spreads God's light to those who need it most.

SET AND ACHIEVE LIFE-CHANGING WELLNESS GOALS

Every great transformation begins with a vision, a goal that inspires action and change. The Bible reminds us of the importance of intentionality and perseverance: "Commit to the Lord whatever you do, and He will establish your plans" (Proverbs 16:3). Setting wellness goals rooted in faith isn't just about improving your physical health—it's about aligning your entire being with God's purpose. These goals are your opportunity to take the biblical principles you've learned and apply them in ways that enrich your life and glorify God.

Steps to Create Faith-Based Wellness Goals

1. **Anchor Goals in Scripture:** Start by asking yourself, "What would God want for my health and life?" Reflect on verses like 1 Corinthians 10:31—"So whether you eat or drink or whatever you do, do it all for the glory of God." Use scripture as a guide to ensure your goals reflect God's will.
2. **Make Them Specific and Achievable:** Avoid vague aspirations like "get healthier." Instead, set clear, actionable goals, such as "spend 10 minutes in prayer every morning" or "replace processed snacks with fresh, God-given foods."
3. **Create a Plan:** Break your goals into manageable steps. For example, if your goal is to honor the Sabbath fully, start by dedicating a few hours each week to rest and worship, gradually building toward a full day.
4. **Pray Over Your Goals:** Invite God into the process, asking for strength, wisdom, and guidance to pursue your goals with His help.
5. **Track Your Progress:** Keep a journal to celebrate victories, reflect on challenges, and stay accountable to the goals you've set.

Living a Life of God-Designed Wellness

As you work toward these goals, remember that the journey is just as important as the destination. Each step you take—whether it's incorporating prayer into your routine, building a healthier diet, or deepening your relationships—is a testament to your commitment to living as God intended. Celebrate progress, no matter how small, and lean on God's strength when setbacks arise. Philippians 1:6 reminds us, "He who began a good work in you will carry it on to completion."

By setting and achieving these goals, you're creating a life that reflects the balance, peace, and vitality of God's healing plan. But more than that, you're becoming a steward of this wisdom, equipped to share it with others. Your journey serves as both a personal transformation and a light to guide others toward biblical wellness.

<u>EMBRACE THE CALL TO BIBLICAL WELLNESS</u>

As you close this book, reflect on how far you've come. You've uncovered truths hidden in scripture—principles for healing, renewal, and abundant living that modern culture often ignores. These aren't just ideas to ponder; they are tools to transform your life and the lives of those around you. God has given you the blueprint for wellness, a sacred plan that encompasses your body, mind, and spirit. Now, it's your turn to live it.

Take what you've learned and commit to making these truths a part of your daily life. Trust that as you align with God's design, you'll experience the fullness of His peace, joy, and vitality. Your journey doesn't end here—it begins. You are now the keeper of hidden healing secrets, empowered to live as God intended and to share this wisdom with the world. May your life shine as a testament to His divine plan for wellness, inspiring others to seek the same transformative truth.

Go forward with faith, and may God bless you abundantly on this journey to wholeness and healing.